Seclusion and Mental Health

A break with the past

Ann Alty

RMN DPSN BA(Hons)
Staff nurse, Mental Health Team, Southport
and Formby Community Health Services NHS Trust,
Merseyside, UK

and

Tom Mason

RMN RNMH RGN BSc(Hons)
Researcher, Ashworth Hospital, Maghull, UK

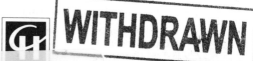

London · Glasgow · Melbourne · Madras

Published by Chapman & Hall, 2–6 Boundary Row, London SE1 8HN, UK

Chapman & Hall, 2–6 Boundary Row, London SE1 8HN, UK

Blackie Academic & Professional, Wester Cleddens Road, Bishopbriggs, Glasgow G64 2NZ, UK

Chapman & Hall GmbH, Pappelallee 3, 69469 Weinheim, Germany

Chapman & Hall Inc., One Penn Plaza, 41st Floor, New York NY 10119, USA

Chapman & Hall Japan, Thomson Publishing Japan, Hirakawacho Nemoto Building, 6F, 1-7-11 Hirakawa-cho, Chiyoda-ku, Tokyo 102, Japan

Chapman & Hall Australia, Thomas Nelson Australia, 102 Dodds Street, South Melbourne, Victoria 3205, Australia

Chapman & Hall India, R. Seshadri, 32 Second Main Road, CIT East, Madras 600 035, India

First edition 1994

© 1994 Chapman & Hall

Phototypeset in 10/12pt Palatino by Intype, London
Printed in Great Britain by Page Bros, Norwich

ISBN 0 412 55230 2

A catalogue record for this book is available from the British Library

Library of Congress Catalog Card Number: 94–70265

♾ Printed on permanent acid-free text paper, manufactured in accordance with ANSI/NISO Z39.48–1992 and ANSI/NISO Z39.48–1984 (Permanence of Paper).

Contents

Preface

Seclusion as a concept is poorly understood and this is reflected in the literature on the topic, particularly from nursing authors. This has led to an emotionally charged altercation rather than academic debate, both within the literature and at conferences. But why bother learning about seclusion at all, particularly as it is used less and less within mental health? We would point out to those sceptical about the value of this book that seclusion is not only of interest as an intervention *per se*, but is valuable in reflecting a shifting ethos within care. For some reason, seclusion has been neglected; we believe that one reason is that it impinges upon widely held myths and beliefs within psychiatric practice. Questioning about seclusion uncovers uncomfortable facts and assumptions concerning the values underpinning today's mental health care approaches. Such uncomfortable questioning is often avoided for safer research pursuits.

Also, we hold that this book is necessary in examining issues pertaining to seclusion practice. There is a gap within nursing knowledge in so far as seclusion is concerned, as our chapter on education upholds. Yet inquiries and litigation have highlighted the fact that seclusion practice must be more clearly understood as an intervention. At present, such understanding is erratic and far from useful in providing a higher standard of care. Practitioners need to make informed decisions regarding seclusion, and this book aims to provide the necessary information on which to base these decisions.

We hope the book will appeal, not only to those in general and forensic psychiatric settings, but also to those in allied caring professions such as mental handicap and social work. It will be a useful text on many courses from Project 2000, post-basic courses and a wide range of diploma and degree courses in health care.

Acknowledgements

In the long, and late, hours worked there are always those who are turned to for assistance and advice. The support comes in many forms, from boosting flagging confidences to more practical organization. Our special thanks are extended to Anne Beadle, Professor Ron Blackburn, Dianne Fawcett, Joyce Hampson, Dave Mercer, Frank Powell and Liz Whybourn for their help, advice, support and encouragement. Also to our respective spouses, Bill and Helen, for tolerating our mood swings as we worked on the manuscript!

1

Introducing seclusion

Tom Mason and Ann Alty

When an individual begins to experience mental illness it is often left to people around him to help. This help may take many forms and guises and, while much of that help is appropriate, great atrocities have taken place in the name of treatment and research. The mentally ill are a marginalized group of people who are often not afforded a voice about how they feel. Indeed, in the rare instances where they are given a voice what they do say may be met with scepticism by the institutions and organizations who care for them. In the past the mentally ill were seen to hold special powers, and could even be burned at the stake as witches due to the fears that their symptoms created in those around them. Since then there has been a subtle shift in emphasis; the mentally ill are now no longer considered to be in touch with spiritual powers which generate awe and fear, but neither are they considered to be in touch with their own rationality. This effectively gives the mentally ill very little credence and leads to other people – some of whom know very little about them – making decisions and choices on their behalf.

Yet, it is argued that times are changing. People who experience mental illness are no longer incarcerated for life in out-of-the-way institutions; the mentally ill are better understood; mental health is about giving choice back to the individual and the old labels no longer stick. Yet, in the midst of these new approaches coercive interventions such as seclusion may be used. Some mentally ill people are locked into a bare room by those who purportedly 'care'. This approach to caring seems to fly in the face of the new era of individualized, holistic and humanistic interventions. Yes, patients are given more choice; yes, professionals are better prepared to listen . . . but professionals still hold tremendous power which continues to be used whenever they deem it necessary, despite well-worded philosophies and mission statements. A sudden change in the modern ethos of caring takes place whenever seclusion is used.

In approaching this book the reader may hold many questions dear in his quest for better understanding. For example, does this coercion mean that the nursing process and modern understanding of mental illness have failed? Why is seclusion so different? Can the concept of overriding another's feelings be considered useful or, indeed, treatment? How is it that one is given power over another because one's perception of that other is held to be more valid and rational? Who ordains this power and who sanctions that medical interpretations override the subjective interpretations of the mentally ill?

There has been, and continues to be, a growing concern regarding seclusion use and abuse which has reached as far as the European Court of Human Rights and the highest courts in America and Britain. The issue has been raised in the House of Commons and the House of Lords, as well as public inquiries which have raised the question of seclusion and have called for its total abolition. The media have sensationalized the scandal of seclusion and the public conscience is duly outraged. Yet despite this huge outcry society itself remains intolerant of the mentally ill. People say that such things ought not to happen and that surely something better should be done. The community may want care for the mentally ill and call for changes, but it is often care on the cheap and done by others, not themselves. This is reflected in murmurings heard by nurses when they divulge that they work with the mentally ill. Often the reaction is, 'I don't know how you do that job' or 'You must be so dedicated . . . ' which demonstrates that the respondent feels that ordinary people simply do not look after such problems for society. It is left to ministering angels or hardened authoritarian figures who have no emotion.

A NEED FOR QUESTIONING

Seclusion has been described as a 'gentle euphemism' (Chamberlin, 1985) which does not accurately explain what actually occurs during the procedure. Indeed, in deciding what to call this book, much debate went into the wording and concern was expressed that the term seclusion would mean nothing to those outside mental health, and would cause problems even for those who claimed to practise seclusion due to the fact that a universal definition is not forthcoming. Many other terms are used to describe what occurs when seclusion is implemented, some of these being 'solitary confinement', 'cell', 'segregation', 'isolation', 'punishment', 'boxed' or 'padded cell'. When approaching a topic such as seclusion, inevitably more questions are going to be raised than answered. Yet some answers are better as questions because this prevents us becoming entrenched in views which do not help the individuals we care for. Seclusion is used less and less in mental illness, yet there are still places designated for seclusion use and there are still times when patients find themselves overridden and locked into a room, for whatever reason.

Seclusion is becoming more and more associated with the negative side of psychiatric care. Other aspects of nursing and medical intervention have evolved and improved, but seclusion remains the same – a locked door. It has been used for centuries and although many dislike the procedure they continue to use it. Yet these negative feelings and approaches do little to help understanding of all the aspects that need to be considered in such an important topic. Seclusion understanding has become as locked away as the procedure itself, and is almost a taboo subject among professionals. We just do not talk about it – or if we are prepared to talk about it we are not prepared to hear any other view but our own. Inevitably we end up talking to ourselves and nothing changes.

This book is an attempt to address this issue. We are, hopefully, unlocking the door on the hidden agendas and effects of seclusion. Only when we understand the complications and concepts associated with seclusion practice can we begin to formulate valuable and expert opinion, and practice which is in keeping with present health care philosophy and approaches. As seclusion is ignored so more opportunity arises for abuse within its practice. Unless these issues are addressed in ways that are viable and valid we are in danger of hiding seclusion away, as we would a bad memory: 'True, it happens but let's try to forget about it'. This 'head-in-the-sand' approach to the problems associated with seclusion usage has already led to well documented inquiries as to its effects, and if it continues will undoubtably afford even more avenues for abuse.

It is necessary, however, at this stage in the book, to differentiate between some terms which are used synonymously within the rhetoric of seclusion terminology. The terms discussed below are often confused with the practice of seclusion when in fact they are often separate issues or misleading descriptions. It is hoped that a clearer understanding of the term seclusion will arise from such discussion. Seclusion is used in many countries and the similarities and differences will also be outlined within this chapter. Finally, we will examine definitional interpretations and discuss the problems in attempting to clearly couch the practice in understandable and cross-cultural terms.

Seclusion and restraint

The term 'seclusion' is often associated with 'restraint'. The two do tend to overlap considerably but seclusion is unique, and therefore worthy of more intense scrutiny; we argue that seclusion is discrete because not only does seclusion restrain certain types of behaviour (usually violence), it effectively removes all social contact. The individual is truly ostracized. Conversely, when a patient is restrained it is still possible to continue social contact and social interaction, whether this be in talking with the patient, touching him or simply sitting with him. Obviously, issues addressed in this text will be applicable and therefore have some bearing on the notion of 'restraints'. However, seclusion is but one aspect of this; effectively, seclusion is a form of situational restraint and deserves to be treated as a unique intervention within mental illness.

Seclusion and 'time out'

Seclusion is also often associated with 'time out' and this has led to problems in definition. Indeed, an article dealing with seclusion practice has, misleadingly, been entitled 'Time Out' (Russell, Hodgkinson and Hillis, 1986). Seclusion and time out are often used synonymously and refer to allowing the patient to lie alone in the seclusion room without the door being locked. In this sense the patient is allowed to 'cool off' and given time to calm down, and should never be associated with the planned care and long-term strategy afforded in time out. It must be stressed that seclusion and time out are entirely different approaches to care. Time out is always part of a planned programme of care, generally with the patient's agreement and understanding (Gibson, 1989). Seclusion, on the other hand, is always an emergency measure to contain and deal with a situation on a short-term basis. There should be clear, planned reasons as to why time out is appropriate for some behaviours, and this should have been decided beforehand as part of a long-term strategy for care.

Seclusion and 'open seclusion'

Another term which may cause confusion and is often used in settings where designated seclusion rooms are available, is 'open seclusion'. Nurses will use this term to avoid classifying the method of segregation used as seclusion identified as a 'locked door' (it also avoids lengthy paperwork and calling doctors out during unsocial hours). 'Open seclusion' refers to the room being used by a patient who is disturbed but with the room left open and unlocked. However, should the patient become extremely disturbed the door is locked and the seclusion period is commenced and recorded from that time. The term, 'open seclusion' is a contradiction, as the nurses and patients know very well that should the patient wish to leave the room the door would be locked, preventing his escape. While opening the door ensures that the patient is not physically locked in the seclusion room, it does not mean that the patient is free to come and go. This 'open seclusion' could well be defined as simply 'seclusion' because the patient is contained within one area against his will, despite the open door. Should patients require restful times alone then 'quiet rooms' would serve the purpose of 'open seclusion'. It would be more appropriate that time spent in the seclusion room which is actually designated for this purpose be termed as a period within seclusion whether or not the door be locked.

Seclusion and 'pindown'

Between 1983 and 1989 a regime of solitary confinement was used in four Staffordshire children's homes to control disturbed children. This regime was termed 'pindown'. It was claimed to be therapeutic, but was eventually highlighted as an abuse of the children in care. In 1991 it was expected that pindown compensation payments would top £2m, the regime being reported as 'intrinsically unethical, unacceptable and unprofessional and a fundamental abuse of human rights' (Dyer, 1991). During pindown children were stripped and denied certain rights from within a locked room as well as being medicated against their will. After discovery of the abuses in the Staffordshire homes similar situations came to light in other areas of the country, and these were sharply criticized. Pindown and other similar techniques were found in almost all childcare sectors (Linton, 1991). Seclusion is not to be confused with pindown, as the children subjected to pindown were not termed 'mentally ill' and pindown was used as part of an intrinsic reward and punishment regime. Seclusion is theoretically used only in caring for those who are mentally ill, and is often an emergency measure in providing safety for either patient or nurse.

CARERS OR CUSTODIANS

Added to this are difficulties due to the fact that concepts of punishment are often associated with seclusion. Western society actually only locks up criminals and the mentally ill, and perceived connections are readily made between the two (and this is accentuated within forensic psychiatry). For this reason alone seclusion needs to be addressed, because being treated like a common criminal when one is merely 'ill' will drastically compound any sense of powerlessness and low self-esteem the patient already perceives, as well as fostering resentment and anger.

Nurses and mental health practitioners are also affected by the fact that seclusion is often associated with punishment. There is a great deal of frustration within nurses, simply due to the fact that their caring role is sometimes viewed by society and their patients as more custodial. This is very stressful for nurses, who enter the profession to care and discover that they are merely containing, and once this custodial approach is adopted towards patients it cannot easily be reversed. It is extremely damaging to therapeutic relationships for a nurse to dominate and manhandle a person one day and attempt to give him autonomy the next! The memory of how that autonomy was overridden the previous day will undoubtably affect any future interaction. In this situation it is easy for the nurse to inform the patient that she is once again supporting him, but the memories that the patient has of being locked away will effectively make a liar of the nurse in so far as the patient is concerned. If this transition from carer to custodian can be avoided it will do much to improve relationships between professionals and patients and prevent unnecessary breakdowns in established relationships.

WORLDWIDE OVERLAP

From the literature around the world it would appear that the responses to violence of the psychiatric patient, particularly in the crisis stage of assault, can be summed up under four headings: seclusion, mechanical restraints, chemical restraints or transfer. These approaches are adopted in one form or another throughout the world (Mason, 1993b).

American literature

By far the greatest number of texts relating to seclusion emanate from America, and in the many cited studies it is apparent that seclusion, restraints and drugs are used, sometimes in isolation and sometimes in combination, to one degree or another throughout America. There is a loud voice of criticism from America (and elsewhere) regarding the use of seclusion, and it is certainly the case that they are concerned over the question of human rights and compulsory treatment. The extent of litigation within American practice regarding seclusion and restraint far exceeds that of other countries. However, we would assume that we in Europe will follow this trend, as seclusion is highlighted as an area readily open to abuse.

Canadian literature

The Canadian articles suggest that, although mechanical restraints are used more often in Canada than in Britain, seclusion itself is used less often (Sreenivasan, 1983). However, as described above, there is also some indication that the terms restraint and seclusion are used interchangeably, which may produce a confounding picture in terms of comparative statistics. In a descriptive study of seclusion Kirkpatrick (1989) reported very similar findings to other studies carried out in America, but concluded that 'Generalisation of the results of this study are limited because the convenience sample was obtained from one institution only'.

Australian literature

The publications located from Australia on seclusion were meagre indeed and any attempt to establish an Australian 'picture' from such a source is susceptible to inaccuracies. Having said that, from one publication (Hafner *et al.*, 1989) it appears that the authors were concerned about similar issues regarding seclusion as are expressed in the general literature by authors from other countries.

European literature

Focusing on Europe, the use of seclusion is heavily overlaid with a complex structure of all methods of restraint. For example, for legislative purposes, seclusion in Poland is encompassed in the much wider term of physical restraint, which also includes emergency measures such as involuntary administration of psychotropic medication; forced feeding; physical (personal) holding; medical treatment or nursing care without the patient's consent. In addition to this Poland also considers seclusion alongside non-consensual means of behaviour control or behaviour modification, as well as force-based actions taken against disturbed patients by police authorities and emergency medical personnel, including ambulance attendants. This understandably confuses the issue when carrying out research into seclusion practice and effects.

In a study on the use of restraints at seven regional psychiatric hospitals which represented a cross-section of such facilities in Poland (Dabrowski, Frydman and Zakowska-Dabrowski, 1986) it was reported that restraint was required on nearly 30% of patients requiring over 14 days' hospitalization.

Brief mention of seclusion was made by the above authors, defining it as ' . . . a treatment or patient control modality which involves the involuntary, indefinite placement of a patient in a locked, secure room, . . . '. However, they eliminated it from their study on the grounds that ' . . . it (seclusion) was found not to be an independent behaviour control modality, it was rarely used and was invariably either preceded or accompanied by other forms of emergency or mechanical restraint'. Interestingly, the above authors also suggested that the decreased use of seclusion in Poland was countered by their increased use of mechanical restraints.

Polish health care workers too are concerned about the issue of abuse in relation to restraint and seclusion. The Polish Mental Health Act specifically defines the requirements for the use of any restraint, and also addresses the therapeutic and behaviour control aspects of its use. The Polish authorities have long been concerned that any treatment facility could be misused for social control purposes, and recognize that the risk of abuse is greatest ' . . . when there is a lack of regulations, laws and internal reviews, or other types of monitoring of its use' (Dabrowski, Frydman and Zakowska-Dabrowski, 1986).

In Switzerland committal of the mentally ill is governed by Article 397 a-f of the Swiss Civil Code (ZGB), but seclusion is regulated by the individual Cantons. In a translated article, Schmied and Ernst (1983) reported a study carried out in the Canton of Zurich and clearly defined seclusion independently of restraint. However, their study was particularly focused upon the considerable overlap between the use of seclusion and the use of involuntary medication.

From the European Regional Council and World Federation for Mental Health conference held in London in November 1991 it was apparent that the overlap between seclusion, restraint and medication was, indeed, widespread. A report from Belgium indicated the use of seclusion in this country, while Denmark claimed not to use seclusion in which patients were left alone but tied to the bed (fixation), always with a nurse beside them.

Holland appeared to use more mechanical restraints than seclusion, with the reverse being the case in Ireland.

Finally, from a tribal society, Laos, in Indochina, who know not of psychiatry nor psychiatrists, there is clear evidence of the use of both seclusion and/or restraints on members of the villages who are deemed *baa* (crazy or insane). The restraints take the form of a series of ropes and chains and the seclusion takes the form of a pit dug in the ground (Westermeyer and Kroll, 1978).

DEFINITIONS

The common understanding of the term seclusion revolves around such notions as peace and tranquillity, with ideas of quiet, hidden beaches and woodlands where people can get away from it all. These connotations are pleasant, with positive overtones. However, to the layperson the seclusion of psychiatric patients conjures up images of 'solitary confinement', 'sensory deprivation', 'padded cells' and 'punishment' and should the individual not know what is meant by the term seclusion (and many do not), the practice would be described in such dubious terms. These images are therefore considered to be negative and speak more of danger and control than peace and tranquillity. Those working in the field of mental health locate the psychiatric use of seclusion between these two extremes, sometimes attempting to define it, at other times not. Many often-cited authors make no attempt to define seclusion in unequivocal terms (Fitzgerald and Long, 1973; Plutchik *et al.*, 1978; Schwab and Lahmeyer, 1979; Binder, 1979; Greenblatt, 1980; Soloff and Turner, 1981; Hodgkinson, 1985; Morrison and Le Roux, 1987), appearing to consider that seclusion is a self-explanatory concept, which may be misinterpreted by lay people but which is understood by those in the allied mental health professions.

Others attempt a loose definition, which also requires an addition of personal experience from the reader if the understanding of the concept is to be clear. For example, 'The confinement of a patient alone in a room, the door which cannot be opened from the inside' (Leopoldt, 1985) and 'The act of temporarily isolating a disturbed patient in a locked room' (Campbell, Shepherd and Falconer, 1982) are definitions which would require further elucidation by some personal knowledge of the experience for there to be a clearer understanding of what seclusion is.

For the purpose of their study Mattson and Sacks (1978) defined seclusion as 'Any patient who required the use of a locked seclusion room at any time during his or her hospitalisation'. Briefer still were Philips and Nasr (1983): 'Placement of a patient in a locked seclusion room', and narrowest of all, 'Locking a patient in a room alone' (Richardson, 1987).

The Royal College of Psychiatrists (1982), referring to the seclusion procedure of patients in the Bethlem Royal and Maudsley Hospitals, define seclusion as ' . . . the containment of a patient alone in a room or other enclosed area from which that patient has no means of egress'. This definition indicates a further relevance, namely, the inability of a secluded patient to gain exit by his or her own free will. This early definition also includes the word 'containment' rather than treatment, which is omitted in the later (1990) definition of seclusion as ' . . . the supervised confinement of a patient specifically placed alone in a locked room for a period of any time of the day or night for the protection of the patient, staff or others from serious harm' (Royal College of Psychiatrists, 1990). The Royal College of Psychiatrists make provision for the use of seclusion as a pre-emptive measure when it is part of a multidisciplinary treatment plan, particularly in relation to the manipulative and disruptive patient.

Strutt *et al.* (1980) raised the issue of the 24-hour recording of seclusion which is pertinent to the special hospitals (as they lock up the majority of their patients each night), and they argue: 'A patient should be regarded to be in seclusion at any time, day or night, when he or she is secluded in a room, the door of which is fastened so that he or she is prevented from leaving the room' (Strutt *et al.*, 1980). Although this definition is lacking in other areas it does incorporate the notion of choice of exit in the phrase 'prevented from leaving the room'.

Kirkpatrick (1989) suggests that a specific place should be demarcated for seclusion use and should be incorporated in the definition, and gives as example ' . . . the placement of a patient, alone, in a specially designated lockable room from which he or she can be observed through a window'.

The Royal College of Nursing (RCN) is less specific in their definition of seclusion as being in a predesignated room and consider that any area in which a patient is confined can be deemed seclusion. They define seclusion as '... the forcible denial of the company of other people by constraint within a closed environment without means of leaving that area' (RCN, 1979). This definition incorporates such factors as the 'social' and 'lack of choice' aspects to seclusion, but omits a rationale.

Thompson's (1986) definition of seclusion as '... a form of situational restraint where the patient is forcibly isolated from other patients in a room, the door of which is locked from the outside' is another example of seclusion existing whenever the door is locked which has obvious implications for the special hospitals, which will be discussed later.

Finally, Gibson (1989) stated: 'Seclusion refers to the removal of an individual, with or without the consent of the individual involved, to a closed/locked environment which he is not permitted to leave'. Although this definition is probably suitable for the majority of psychiatric establishments it remains inappropriate for the special hospitals, as it would refer to all patients for most of the time due to the fact that patients are locked into their own rooms each night.

USE OF THE TERM SECLUSION IN THIS BOOK

As discussed previously, we feel it is important to recognize that seclusion can be defined separately from the concept of restraint. However, adding a further definition to the already complicated definitions described above would cause even more confusion. Nonetheless, there are some general understandings of the word as used within mental health which accurately describe what seclusion is.

The previously described definitions do, however, highlight certain common understandings about the situation of seclusion. In a study by Mason (1992) it was discovered that there were seven fundamental components, with no definition incorporating all seven: place (i.e. a designated area for seclusion); social isolation; egress; compulsion (i.e. moving, against the will of the patient, to another area); time (duration of seclusion); rationale (reasons for seclusion); and finally establishment (felt by Mason not to necessarily be part of any definition).

We would uphold that seclusion involves a locked door and that the door is locked by someone other than the patient. Also it is important to realize that seclusion ensures that all direct social contact is withdrawn from the patient. Additionally, it is understood that seclusion involves force being used by carers towards those they care for. When a patient asks to go into seclusion it is debatable as to whether seclusion is the appropriate intervention. We do not feel that placing a patient in a seclusion room when he asks can actually be considered to be seclusion in its purest sense.

LEVEL OF DEBATE

Mason (1991) identified differing levels of debate concerning the use of seclusion. For example, official reports (20) from governmental, professional and academic departments reported much concern about the use and abuse of seclusion, and generally speaking the debate revolved sensibly around the practical issues and procedural difficulties. Research studies, literature reviews and articles with at least one research component (79) revealed attempts at academic approaches in the understanding of this complex issue, and involved descriptive, analytical and interpretive texts on seclusion. There were a number of related articles (84) covering such issues as restraints, violence, sensory deprivation and nursing care of the secluded patient. Finally, there were the quasi-ideological pronunciations, from a supposed moral framework from both sides of the argument, mainly from nurses.

It is well understood that seclusion is an extremely emotive topic. Its proponents claim that those opposed to it are unable to provide a realistic alternative other than increased medication and physical restraints. They argue that those condemning its use from a safe distance, far removed from the areas in which nurse–patient interactions occur, provide little but vacuous and inane ideological statements. They maintain that those opposed to its use without the support of alternatives and/or resources are failing in their duty to provide a healthy and safe working environment and are, in reality, abusing ward-based nurses as expendable items to be injured and possibly discarded.

However, those who argue for the abolition of seclusion maintain that seclusion continues because of staff fears of losing control, of losing power, and of losing dominance. They argue that those who believe in its use are traditionalists, custodians and intransigent to change, and that they have no place in modern psychiatry. They believe seclusion is an archaic, outmoded and punitive means of controlling disturbed behaviours.

It is, of course, not always as clear-cut as this. There are many whose beliefs regarding seclusion lie somewhere in the middle of the foregoing arguments. In any event, it is right that we should be concerned about the use of seclusion but this concern should lead us on a quest to understand the complexities of the issue, and urge us to investigate realistic approaches to the management of disturbed behaviour.

THREE APPROACHES TO SECLUSION

In this short section we would like to briefly outline three themes that will be developed more fully throughout the book, and hope that all those interested in the seclusion of the mentally ill will find them useful for reflective thinking.

From the literature reviewed it became apparent that there was often a large emotional content evident in many of the texts, even from articles that purported to undertake empirical research studies. There appeared to be a clear division between literature based on personal views and literature based on genuine research studies of one method or another. However, there was also a clear delineation within the personal views category between what may be called the constructionists and the quasi-religious ideologists. Therefore, these three will be described below and are categorized as: (1) personal view constructionist, (2) personal view quasi-religious ideologist, and (3) systematic research. Those for and against seclusion are identifiable within all three of the above categories.

Personal view constructionist

Those articles which we would place within the personal view constructionist category include, for example, Gutheil (1978) who sets out his personal views in support of seclusion while constructing a lucid theoretical base and providing a clear conceptual framework. Similarly, but arguing strongly against the use of compulsory interventions, Szasz (1978) located the notion of coercive psychiatry within the realms of social control, once again producing a conceptual framework on which his personal views are hung. Although these personal views are opposed, they are helpful to the debate on seclusion as they are based on the construction of underlying concepts which throw light on the subject and aid the debate.

Personal view quasi-religious ideologists

Personal views from a quasi-religious ideological base are in the main from the nursing literature on seclusion. They may be a reflection on nurse education (discussed in Chapter 8) and the popular tradition of relating the work of nursing to the religious notion of its being a vocation, with the dominant (and often bigoted) value systems of right and wrong, good and evil. For example, from the often-cited text of Pilette (1978) arguing against the 'tyranny of seclusion', we hear an emotional plea on behalf of the patients, who 'from the abyss of their mind they cry out in terror for love and caring'. Pilette does not cite any reference or research in support of this emotive view but her expressed concern is often cited as if it were valid research evidence. Even more poignantly, arguments have been put forward that seclusion and isolation may be places of 'last sanctuary' and possibly the ' . . . lesser of several *evils*' (Miller, 1992) (emphasis added). Although such strong personal views are important in motivating change and demonstrating values, they are at best less than useful in academic studies and at worst serve only to confuse and confound the seclusion issue. In fact, using these emotive pleas instead of valid research evidence does much to demonstrate the immaturity of the nursing profession. While such emotive expressions indicate that change is wanted, they do nothing to facilitate such change as they fail to provide strong, research-based practical solutions to the seclusion debate. The emotional response is important, but care must be taken in assessing the evidence upon which the response is based. Such emotional pleas often omit factual analysis.

Systematic research

Fortunately, the third and final category is increasingly taking the dominant position in the literature, much of which is based on empirical research studies that produce quantitative and qualitative data for analysis and interpretation, and do so without recourse to emotional ramblings. One excellent example is

Soliday (1985), with a comparison of patient and staff attitudes towards seclusion, with each group believing seclusion to be negative and positive, respectively. Another outstanding example is the work carried out by Gerlock and Solomons (1983). In Britain much work has been carried out by P. Morrison (1990) and Mason (1992), who have set the scene for valuable research findings but have only really begun to explore the neglected topic of seclusion. Much work is yet to be done.

There are many approaches to the study of seclusion and we have sought to collate material and research findings from a large range of sources. Some of the material described has never been published before and is based on our own research. Seclusion is a complicated procedure which has been affected by history, education, culture, medicine and law. It is hoped that addressing these issues will help any student of psychiatry and psychiatric nursing to grasp the concepts and formulate their own thinking based on factual analysis rather than emotive reactions. In understanding more about seclusion and the concepts and constructs surrounding its usage, it is further hoped that the patients we care for will reap the benefit of improved approaches to care in what is undoubtably a most vulnerable episode in their lives.

his madness by letting him see many different faces will be avoided.' (Soranus Of Ephesus, 5?? AD)

Soranus goes on to describe in detail how servants ought to interact with the patient and recommends massage as a way of soothing the patient. He also points out that patients ought to be bound if they become too excitable.

Gibson (1989) and others point out that the above was an early recommendation for the use of seclusion; however, it appears from the translation of his work that social contact is never withdrawn from the patient and the patient is never locked away alone. This therefore does not fit into our understanding of seclusion as implemented by today's practitioners, where locked doors and withdrawn human contact are commonplace.

It was Egypt and the Middle East that led the way in providing hospitals for the care of the mentally ill. Hospitals were known to be put aside entirely for the care of the insane in Arabian cities around the years 700–1200 AD (Maddison, Day and Leabeater, 1975). Spanish monks began treating the mentally ill with 'moral treatments' and claimed to have a high success record long before others conceived of this method (similar to that of Tukes and Pinel described below (Seguin, 1866).) Spain began building hospitals for the insane during the 15th century, but the first British institution designated to take care of the 'insane' was at Bethlehem (also known as Bethlem or Bedlam) in London. A man named Simon Fitzmary founded the Priory of St Mary of Bethlehem in 1247 in Bishopsgate. It is recorded that by 1403 sick people were sent there, and this included six men who were insane. Bethlem was soon established as a place where the acutely insane could be sent. However, other hospitals are also known to have set aside beds for the insane. For example, Trinity Hospital in Salisbury, established in the 14th century, allocated 30 beds for the sick where the mad were kept safe (Allderidge, 1978).

By the 18th century Bethlem remained the only public institution entirely given over to care of the insane, alongside other private 'madhouses', and those sent there were not covered by policy or laws to look after their interests. Once incarcerated in a building such as Bethlem the insane were never afforded a visit by a physician or clergy, and relatives were kept away if at all possible. The exceptions to this were paying visitors, who were charged twopence to watch the insane at Bethlem at the turn of the 18th century. The insane were viewed as 'sport' by the population, and were often intimidated into a frenzy by their keepers if they did not perform adequately for the paying visitors (Glover, 1984).

EARLY TREATMENTS

Early attempts at treatment for the insane were shrouded in superstitious theory and moral judgement. A leading figure was a man named Burton (1576–1639), who basically felt that it was personal sin or the work of the devil that brought about insanity; however, he also held that there were certain predisposing or contributory factors, which he classified into six 'non-natural things': bad air, the retention of bodily excretions (constipation etc.), bad diet and lack of sleep, too much or too little exercise and emotional disturbances. (Burton *The Anatomy Of Melancholy* 1676, cited in Jones, 1955). This view was held to a greater or lesser degree by those caring for the insane during the following century, and various approaches to 'treatment' were founded on Burton's theories. The working classes often believed that the insane were witches, inflicting torture and other primitive methods of 'treatment' on them in an attempt to effect a cure. There was no standardization of medical qualifications and it was left to untrained or minimally trained 'apothecaries' to provide care and treatment for the mentally ill (Copeman, 1967). These apothecaries were trained by senior physicians to concoct simple herbal remedies and carry out minor surgical techniques popular at the time, such as bleeding (where veins were opened to release blood and thus, it was hoped, the illness) and purging, whereby strong emetics and laxatives were given to patients to rid them of bodily excretions. Another method of 'treating' the insane was to carry out trephining, where bore holes were made with simple tools into the patient's skull to enable the 'bad humors', which were believed to affect the brain, to escape. Needless to say, these apothecaries administered their treatments in very crude and intuitive ways which often had no real value. In fact, procedures such as trephining, purges and blood letting had severe outcomes for the patients involved, and it was not unusual for them to die from their treatment. These treatments were also carried out in America, where in 1783 a leading doctor, Benjamin Rush, advised that the insane should be beaten and insulted regularly (Maddison, Day and eater, 1975). Rush also developed the 'tranquillizer chair', ich was used to restrain the insane and give easy access for ood letting and other treatments. On 24 September 1810 Rush wrote to the Pennsylvania Hospital Managers making recommendations for better care and sanitary conditions for his patients. Among these recommendations was one that reads: 'That small and solitary buildings be erected at a convenient distance from the west wing of the Hospital for the reception of patients in the high and distracted state of madness . . .' (Rush, 1810). This was largely in order not to disturb the other patients in his care, but seems to be a recommendation for a drastic use of seclusion.

Treatment at this time also relied heavily on controlling the insane by physical weakening and fear. The physical weakening relied much on the same 'treatments' described above and often took the form of blood letting, purges, vomits or blisters (applying heat in various forms to the skin to raise a water blister). Sometimes leeches were applied to draw blood out, and sometimes the patients were actually physically denied food in order for them to become malnourished and therefore weak and less aggressive. It was felt strongly at the time that making the patient fearful was useful in control (Rosen, 1968). Patients were therefore threatened and abused, sometimes by overt threats but often in the name of 'treatment'. For example, one of these treatments was named 'the bath of surprise', where the patient was plunged suddenly through a wooden trapdoor into a cold bath. Another was named the 'revolving chair', into which the unfortunate person was strapped and spun until he screamed for mercy and eventually passed out. Combined with these treatments were the use of restraints such as chains, shackles, straitwaistcoats and darkened rooms. The conditions under which the insane were kept were extremely basic, with near nakedness and straw bedding reported at Bethlem; but in other areas where the insane were kept, such as gaols or Bridewells, complete nakedness and bare floors were reported.

There was, at this time, a strong belief in discipline and it is to be noted that one of these disciplines included solitary confinement in a darkened room for 'mischievous conduct' (Jones, 1955). With this in mind it is not difficult to understand how seclusion has sometimes been associated with punishment of the individual.

EARLY BRITISH LAW AND CARE OF THE MENTALLY ILL

(Space does not permit a detailed examination of all public general statutes concerned with care of the mentally ill. A list of these is included at the end of the chapter for reference.)

By the 17th century the insane were still offered no legal rights nor protection under British law. The Poor Law, based on the Act of 1601, stated that 'unpaid overseers of the poor were to raise money weekly or otherwise by taxation in each parish for the relief of its own paupers' (Jones, 1955), and the insane were thus looked after under these auspices. The insane were also disseminated into various organizations to contain them, depending largely on their behaviour. Thus, at the turn of the 18th century the insane may have been confined in 'Bridewells' (houses of correction for those committing minor offences such as 'wandering abroad'), or may have been found in gaol due to more serious misdemeanours. Alternatively, the insane could be kept in workhouses. Many of these institutions eventually segregated the acutely insane, but provided them with little sustenance or hygiene. Often the insane were kept in their own homes and were frequently chained and restrained inside sheds and outhouses, or under the stairs and in cellars. In middle-class families the insane might be given their own room with attendants, and it was not unusual for them to be hidden away, so that people were not even aware of their existence. A graphic description of this is given in the novel *Jane Eyre*, where Jane describes being taken to see the insane wife of her employer:

'He lifted the hangings from the wall, uncovering the second door; this, too, he opened. In a room without a window, there burnt a fire, guarded by a high and strong fender, and a lamp suspended from the ceiling by a chain. Grace Poole bent over the fire, apparently cooking something in a saucepan. In the deep shade, at the further end of the room, a figure ran backwards and forwards. What it was, whether beast or human being, one could not, at first sight, tell: it grovelled, seemingly, on all fours; it snatched and growled like some strange wild animal: but it was covered with clothing; and a quantity of dark, grizzled hair, wild as a mane, hid its head and face.' (Bronte, 1847)

Because of all these differing Acts and organizations that gave custody to the insane, management of the insane was not recognized as a separate need nor did they warrant specialized treatment other than containment.

18TH CENTURY LEGISLATION

Thus it seemed that the insane were viewed with superstition by the working class, with moral condemnation by the church (they believed that human misery was a result of personal sin) and with ignorance by the apothecaries and keepers who tended them. It has been argued that the beginning of segregation of the mentally ill was the result of a mature capitalist market economy and its associated commercialism (Scull, 1989). Indeed, it has been pointed out that 'The secularisation of ideas about insanity and of psychological healing was an aspect of the governing classes' response to the political and religious conflicts of the seventeenth century' (MacDonald, 1980).

In 1744 direct mention was made of the 'violently insane' in an Act dealing with vagrancy. This brought the plight of the insane into the political arena for the first time. The ensuing legislation regulating care of the insane proved tardy in arriving, and in 1774 an Act made provisions for madhouses only to be managed by those approved and licensed by the commissioners, who were subsequently responsible to parliament for their decisions. The commissioners had important responsibilities: they were to be informed of new admissions to the madhouses and were to visit and make inspections regularly; it was also their responsibility to ensure that no-one was unlawfully detained, and that those who were there were treated with dignity and kindness. Unfortunately the act was 'so ineffectual that it remained almost a dead letter' (Jones, 1955), saying nothing about medical supervision, overcrowding, restraint or deliberate brutality of treatment. The commissioners under the Act of 1774 gave evidence to a select committee on the madhouses they supervised, in both 1815 and 1816. Many patients remained chained and unnecessarily restrained and it was reported that they were often starved, so that they presented no management problems for the carers.

CHANGING ATTITUDES TOWARDS MENTAL ILLNESS

In the mid-18th century public prisons continued to house the insane. A major influence on bringing about change in Britain's prisons was John Howard (1726–1791), who became sheriff of Bedford County in 1773. He was appalled at conditions in British prisons and during his campaign visited all prisons in England and Ireland, as well as most European prisons. He found the insane were locked away without treatment in extremely poor conditions and diseases were widespread, as was corruption by the keepers. Change was slow, but steps were taken to improve matters due to this man's work (Goshen, 1967).

In the late 18th century George III became ill with what was then termed 'insanity'. As King George was popular this ensured that the general public no longer perceived the onset of insanity with quite the same amount of superstition. As George III experienced times when he was well he was afforded support and retained his position, which was unusual for people felt to be 'insane'. It was around this time that a few socially concerned individuals founded more sympathetic institutions to care for the insane. These included St Lukes, London (founded 1751); Manchester Lunatic Hospital (founded 1766) and the York Retreat (founded in June 1792). The York Retreat was founded by a tea merchant named William Tuke, a strong Quaker who sought to provide care which facilitated health and emotional support for the people sent there. Good food and exercise were high on the agenda and large exercise corridors were built to allow the irritable patient to walk around at will. This particular approach was named 'mild treatment' by those at the Retreat and later came to be known as 'moral treatment' as it relied heavily on education and approaches that respected individuals as being able to control their own behaviour.

19TH CENTURY LEGISLATION

The new madhouses did much to influence 19th century legislation. Much of the care offered at these centres was based on moral rather than medical reforms, and included good food and basic rights to exercise for the restless patients. The County Asylums Act of 1808 (known as Wynn's Act) was based on both evangelicalism and radicalism, and less on medical intervention, and resulted in the founding of County Asylums for the care of the insane. However, this was not welcomed politically when further Bills to designate an inspectorate to preserve the rights of lunatics in asylums met with opposition from the House of Lords. At the third reading, Lord Eldon, the then Lord Chancellor, stated: 'There could not be a more false humanity than over humanity with regards to persons afflicted with insanity' (cited by Jones, 1960). Eldon felt that any attempt to improve conditions for the insane reflected social unrest and was to be deplored as liberal sentiment. However, the County Asylums Act and the Madhouse Act, both of 1828, moved legislation and thinking forward.

However, Jones (1955) points out that by 1832 there were still five different auspices under which the insane could be held in Britain: private 'madhouses' under Gordon's Act and the Act of 1832; County Asylums, under the second of Gordon's Acts; workhouses, controlled by local authorities; Bethlem; and finally, 'single lunatics' in private homes. These five provisions necessitated five distinct systems of administration: the Lord Chancellor's Office administered the private madhouses; the County Asylums were controlled by the Home Department; it was left to local authorities or Poor Law Commissioners to supervise the workhouses; there was no legal supervision at all for those in Bethlem; and those kept at home were cared for under the Madhouses Act of 1828. However, not everyone declared when they were looking after the insane and it was extremely difficult to trace those kept individually. There was no coordination of care between these departments and thus a cohesive understanding of care was not available to help cope with the mentally ill in British society. The County Asylums Act and the Madhouse Act of 1828 did, however, pave the way for a better approach to care, which was shared and developed by a number of people.

In Britain, Dr John Conolly visited the asylum in Lincoln, influenced by the work of Pinel and run by Drs Gardiner, Hill and Charlesworth. Conolly then took the practice of non-restraint into what was then Britain's largest asylum, having 1000 beds in Middlesex in the year 1839 (Crammer, 1990). Conolly was known to be a 'sentimental humanist unfitted for the detached and painstaking work of medical research' (Jones, 1955). He had studied in Edinburgh and enjoyed a good reputation in medical practice; however, his fellow practitioners were suspicious of his changes in approach to caring for the insane. It was Conolly who gave great publicity and debate to lack of restraints, yet he too supported the use of seclusion as a means of controlling extreme violence and agitation. He wrote: 'That salutory exclusion of cause of excitement from an already irritated brain, has been so unjustly stigmatized as solitary imprisonment' (Conolly, 1856 cited by Hodgkinson, 1985). Hodgkinson also points out that Conolly 'Acknowledged that the spirit with which seclusion was enforced was crucial, and that if it included anger, contempt, punishment or neglect, it reproduced the evils of the mechanical restraint he abhorred' (Hodgkinson, 1985).

Conolly's philosophy made a great impression in America, where practitioners began introducing their own changes.

Another doctor who supported the non-use of mechanical restraint was Samuel Gaskell, who became superintendent of Lancaster Moor Asylum in 1840. At this time, Lancaster Moor was the second largest asylum in the country, and when he was appointed Gaskell immediately began to release patients. Gaskell left Lancaster Moor Asylum 9 years later and, sadly, his work was neglected in his absence, which highlights the fact that the care of patients relied heavily on the beliefs and expertise of the people in charge of the hospital. There was often difficulty in recruiting nurses and attendants who upheld this view, but overall the change did gradually take place, albeit at a slow rate, as more and more people came to believe in the importance of release for the insane in the County Asylums. Lord Shaftsbury became a great political reformer on behalf of the paupers and mentally ill in 19th century Britain and he advocated and supported the Acts of Parliament that sought to improve the conditions and understanding of the mentally ill.

CARE OF THE MENTALLY ILL IN AMERICA AND EUROPE

The work at the York Retreat became known in the United States. Samuel Tuke (1784–1857), grandson of William Tuke who founded the Retreat, wrote a book entitled *Description of the Retreat*, outlining the theory and methods used there. Shortly afterwards the Bloomingdale Asylum in New York, the Hartford Retreat, Frankford Asylum and the McLean Hospital near Boston were founded based on the innovative work in York (Goshen, 1967).

It was possible for Americans to force their wives and children into asylums without legal or medical agreement, and this was abused, as the fascinating account of an ex-patient, Mrs Packard, demonstrates. In her account she describes in detail her abduction from home one morning in June 1860, being taken on the wish of her husband to an asylum (Packard, 1885). The description of filth and injustice she was made to endure as an 'insane' woman, which she published on her eventual release, did much to bring about changes in civil rights in America.

As in Britain, the insane were often segregated into almshouses and county hospitals as well as asylums. A lady named Dorothea Lynde Dix (1802–1887) saw the more advantageous approach to care provided at the Boston Asylum and argued strongly that local control of asylums was failing and that state-owned institutions would afford much better, standardized care. At least 30 state hospitals were built following her recommendations. Miss Dix's campaign demonstrates once again that certain reforms at this time were more to do with public moral concern than major improvements in treatments, as she was simply a schoolmistress from Boston. In an address to the Massachusetts Legislature in 1843, she described situations for the insane, including the fact that they were placed in 'cages, closets, stalls, pens! Chained, naked, beaten with rods, and lashed into obedience' (Dix, 1843). There appears to have been a method of auctioning insane people along with paupers to the lowest bidders (possibly to raise funds), and this is also described by Dix in her address.

The superintendent of the Pennsylvania hospital, Thomas Kirkbride (1809–1883), describes seclusion and uses the term much as we would today. He argues that seclusion and restraint are 'evils of no trifling magnitude' as they 'tend to produce a relaxation of vigilance' (Kirkbride, 1854). He goes on to state that seclusion and restraint can become too readily used by attendants, who 'regard them as their grand reliance in every emergency', thus laying aside 'less objectionable' approaches to dealing with violence (Kirkbride, 1854). Kirkbride also recommended that restraints be used over and above seclusion, as he felt that prolonged seclusion resulted in bad habits which were 'most unfortunate for the future prospects of the patient' (Kirkbride, 1854).

However, not all psychiatrists and reformers in America saw the moral approach to care as useful. A major figure in arguing against these treatments was John Gray, who was editor of the *Journal of Insanity* from 1854 to 1866. It is stated that he did much to bring about the poor custodial care in American institutions, and he refused to allow any articles on moral treatments to be published in his journal, which led other psychiatrists to follow his example (Goshen, 1967).

It was post-revolution Paris that saw the first changes in approach to the care of the insane in France. A doctor named Philippe Pinel was in charge of a hospital in Paris and, with his senior male attendant, nurse Jean-Baptiste Pussin, he released 40 patients from their chains and restraints in 1798. He was said to have been influenced greatly by the work at the York Retreat in England. This was the first time in medical history that previously detained patients were released and given occupation, and it was carried into Britain by Drs Gardner, Hill and Charlesworth, who brought this approach into practice at their asylum in Lincoln and further developed it until the whole asylum functioned without restraints. It is extremely interesting to note that Pinel continued to use seclusion, and stated that 'strait waistcoats, superior force and seclusion for a limited time, are the only punishments inflicted' at the hospital Bicetre, where he worked. There is never any mention in early documentation of seclusion being a treatment method. The locking up of a patient away from social contact is always described as 'containment' or 'punishment'. Also, Pinel still advocated locking patients in darkened rooms at times. He wrote: 'Close confinement, solitude, darkness and a spare diet, may no doubt be incurred occasionally, and for a short time, as a punishment for the improper demeanour of maniacs' (Pinel, 1806).

Austria was also making progress in caring for the mentally ill, although much is made of restraining the 'overexcited will'. Ernst Von Feuchtersleben (1806–1849) was the first notable psychiatrist in Austria; he wrote a major publication entitled *The Principles of Medical Psychology*, in which he describes using darkness, repose and solitude as useful ways of controlling the will of his patients (Goshen, 1967).

DEVELOPMENT OF FORENSIC PSYCHIATRY

The 'McNaughten Rule' was established in 1843 by the House of Lords after a murder trial where the defendant, McNaughten, was accused of murdering a politician. It transpired that McNaughton was under the delusion that this politician was Robert Peel, and that it was in fact Robert Peel whom he had attempted to murder. The trial debated his ability to comprehend what crime he had committed, in view of his mental illness, and a rule was established indicating that no-one can be held responsible for a crime he did not understand. From this, great interest arose in establishing when criminal responsibility occurs and how the accused ought to be dealt with (Goshen, 1967).

Wilhelm Griesinger (1817–1868) became one of the most influential psychiatrists in Germany at this time. Griesinger began to take an interest in the statistics of illnesses in Europe. He made some interesting observations about prisoners and their incidence of mental illness, and asked: 'The question still remains unsolved, and probably in the present state of our knowledge it cannot be solved. What is the influence of the various new systems of punishment on the mental health of the criminal?' (Griesinger, 1845). A fellow German, Johann Ludwig Casper, published a book entitled *A Handbook of The Practice Of Forensic Medicine* in 1845, which won him great influence in the development of forensic psychiatry.

In the USA Isaac Ray (1807–1881) was carrying out valuable work in forensic psychiatry at the mental hospital in Maine (Goshen, 1967).

EARLY MEDICATION AND SECLUSION

Sedatives and hypnotic drugs such as bromides, chloral and paraldehyde were introduced in the mid to late 19th century, and were welcomed for controlling severely disturbed patients. Yet even with new technological developments and the new policy reforms seclusion was advocated as a form of treatment for the violent or extremely agitated, as records from the York Retreat clearly demonstrate (Jones, 1955). Each ward was allocated a padded cell and the 1890 Lunacy Act ensured that nurses were not allowed to seclude without a superintendent signing it in a special book (Crammer, 1990). It is interesting to note that there has been no direct statutory basis for seclusion since that Act of 1890 in Britain.

DEVELOPMENT OF PSYCHIATRIC NURSING

The psychiatric nurse (or attendants) had much to do with implementing change in the care of the mentally ill. It was Conolly who brought great academic credence to the practice of releasing patients, and in 1856 suggested that nurses for the mentally ill needed professional training. In 1891 examinations for mental nurses began in Britain on a national scale; interestingly, this was implemented many years before general nursing examinations, The General Nursing Council and state registration only beginning in 1920 and the two qualifications remaining distinct until the NHS Act of 1946.

POSTWAR LEGISLATION IN BRITAIN

The British Mental Health Act 1959 heralded new appraisals of the rights of the insane. This was largely due to reliable psychotropic medication providing an alternative means of stabilizing patients. Doors were unlocked and the rights of the patients were theoretically safeguarded. It was, however, generally held that seclusion was still necessary and 'good for the patient', but some began to question the whole practice of psychiatry and strongly criticized the western model of psychiatric care (Szasz, 1962; Goffman, 1968; Laing, 1985). The 'antipsychiatrists', as they became known, heralded a whole new philosophical and moral thinking which sought to dismantle what they saw as the farce of psychiatric care, but practice changed little, as these critics provided no future structure for changing care. However, their observations brought valid epistemological and ontological questioning about the nature of mental disease and its treatment, as well as bringing moral reasoning more into the foreground (Wulff, Pederson and Rosenberg, 1990). The 1983 Mental Health Act further placed legal rights into the hands of patients and their advocates, and continued to encourage debate surrounding seclusion. In the 1970s, 1980s and 1990s nursing literature began to reflect this changing ethos of care, and some writers related this to the practice of seclusion. Some areas even began to practise 'non-seclusion policies' (Kingdon and Bakewell, 1988). Organizations such as MIND (National Association for Mental Health) became more involved in commenting on psychiatric care, and nursing bodies such as the United Kingdom Central

Council (UKCC) developed codes of conduct (UKCC, 1984; 1992a) which dealt directly with the ethical aspects of nursing. The UKCC was established under the Nurses, Midwives and Health Visitors Act of 1979, and was expected to maintain an up-to-date register of all practising nurses, midwives and health visitors, and to provide a monitoring system of practice-related issues. Finally, in 1991 the Patients' Charter was developed, to be introduced on April 1 the following year, and this again encouraged practitioners and service users to consider ethical dilemmas related to practice. The current legislation is considered at length in Chapter 5.

FINAL OBSERVATIONS

It is difficult to ascertain exactly what influences change in psychiatric practice, whether it be politics or industry, individual pioneers or religious reforms such as the Reformation. What is apparent, however, is that approaches to care have, to some extent, altered. Unfortunately, seclusion continues to be practised without supporting evidence that it is useful, largely because it has been practised historically all over the world. It is apparent, however, that research concerning the social, political and historical contexts of psychiatry (including seclusion practice) is wholly unsatisfactory in establishing definite clues as to reasons for these changes in care for the mentally ill. To simply state that people began to understand more about psychology is not enough; to point out that political unrest or religious fervour affected change does not explain how this occurred. Psychiatry is deeply embedded in sociological, political and ideological developments within society, and cannot be viewed simply as a chronological order of events and people who brought them about. The history of mental illness in England is incomplete at present, and the historical influences are extremely important in understanding current approaches to care. In a paper that attempts to demonstrate that insanity is 'very much a matter for the historian', MacDonald (1980) points out that there is much research yet to be done before a 'satisfactory history of insanity' is completed. He concludes: 'Historians who undertake that challenging task will not be neglecting the reality of the past' (MacDonald, 1980).

SUMMARY OF BRITISH LEGISLATION CONCERNING CARE OF
THE MENTALLY ILL, 1601–1983

Poor Law Act 1601
Vagrancy Act 1744
Act For Regulating Private Madhouses 1774
Criminal Lunatics Act 1800
County Asylums Act 1808
County Asylums Act 1828
Madhouse Act 1828
Lunatics Act 1832
Poor Law Amendment Act 1834
Criminal Lunatics Act 1838
Criminal Lunatics Act 1840
Lunatics Property Act 1842
Lunatic Asylums Act 1842
Lunatics Act 1845
Lunatic Asylums And Pauper Lunatics Act 1845
Lunacy Regulation Act 1853
Lunatics Care And Treatment Amendment Act 1853
Lunatics Asylums Amendment Act 1853
Lunatics Law Amendment Act 1862
Lunatics Law Amendment Act 1889
Lunacy (Consolidation) Act 1890
Mental Deficiency Act 1913
Mental Deficiency Act 1927
Mental Treatment Act 1930
National Health Service Act 1946
Mental Health Act 1959
Mental Health Act 1983

3

Literature review

Tom Mason

In a recent project one of the authors (Mason, 1991) was commissioned by the Special Hospitals Service Authority (SHSA) for England and Wales to carry out research into the use of seclusion, and part of this project involved an extensive review of the literature from around the world.

The professional disciplines reviewed during the project included nursing, medicine, psychology, sociology, social work, social anthropology and public health. The procedure involved carrying out searches of national and international indexes, abstracts, journals, bibliographies and reference lists, from published sources as well as unpublished dissertations from universities. The search also included governmental publications from a number of departments.

Computer searches were undertaken on DHSS (Department of Health and Social Security), MEZZ (Medline), EMZZ/EMED (Excerpta Medica), PSYCINFO (Psychological Abstracts and Allied Fields) and SOCA (Sociological Abstracts) databases. These articles were then divided into five main categories, and although there was often an overlap between the categories seclusion remained the central theme. The categories and number of references (which have been updated at the time of writing) can be seen in Figure 3.1.

A subdivision of the seclusion articles into the following areas was found to be useful, although it must be remembered that some articles overlapped considerably.

1. Facts, statistics and research findings
2. Theory and interpretation

Type of Articles	Freq
SECLUSION	91
RESTRAINT AND SECLUSION	11
VIOLENCE AND SECLUSION	30
ALTERNATIVES AND TIME-OUT	9
SELECTED RELATED ARTICLES	23

Figure 3.1 Number of published articles relating to seclusion

3. Methods and procedures
4. Opinions, beliefs and points of view
5. Anecdotes, clinical impressions and narrations.

From the literature reviewed several themes emerged in which to situate the information.

DEFINITIONS

It was found that seclusion was popularly linked to solitary confinement and punishment, and that there were many terms used to describe the practice. These included isolation, shuttered room, quiet room, unfurnished room, protective room, cleared room, suite of secure rooms and padded cell.

As was pointed out in Chapter 1, some authors make no attempt to define seclusion, which suggests that workers in the field of mental health have a common understanding of the term without the need to make this explicit. Other authors did attempt to define seclusion, for example Leopoldt (1985): 'the confinement of a patient alone in a room, the door of which cannot be opened from the inside', and Richardson (1987): 'locking a patient in a room alone'. Unfortunately, such definitions, by being limited to merely a question of geography and egress, do not provide a fuller meaning of seclusion, which leaves the definition found wanting.

The literature review highlighted seven fundamental components to the definition of seclusion (Mason, 1992):

1. Place
2. Social isolation
3. Egress
4. Compulsion
5. Time
6. Rationale
7. Establishment in which it takes place.

It is the establishment, or institution, that gives seclusion practice its cultural context, and without this being included it will remain unclear as to what seclusion means.

SECLUSION AND TIME OUT

It would appear, both from the literature reviewed and from a number of visits to various hospitals and units, that seclusion and time out are often used interchangeably, which is an incorrect use of the terminology. The term time out is misused as representing a period of rest, or time to 'sleep it off', i.e. a cooling-down period. Although both rationales are appropriate strategies for preventing a deterioration in a psychiatric emergency they are not, strictly speaking, time out.

Time out is part of the application of the scientific analysis of behaviour known as behaviour modification, and should always be part of a behaviour modification programme. The term time out refers to time out from positive reinforcement, and includes one of three elements. First, the removal of a positive reinforcer for a specified period of time immediately following the presentation of an undesirable behaviour. In this use of time out it is the external positive reinforcer that is removed, and not the patient. A second form of time out is the partial removal of a patient from the source of the positively reinforcing stimulus, but not from its environment. The third type is the complete removal of the patient from the positive reinforcing environment (Linkenhoker, 1974).

Unless the use of time out is clearly rooted in an identified behaviour modification programme, 'the procedure of isolating a patient from his fellows is an example of seclusion and it is misleading to name it otherwise' (Thorpe, 1980).

GEOGRAPHICAL SPACE AND FURNISHINGS

The literature reviewed revealed a surprising consensus regarding both the descriptions of seclusion rooms and the extent of furnishings provided.

Most authors agree that the seclusion room should be located near the centre of the ward milieu activity, but also suggest that it should afford the patient a degree of privacy. If the seclusion room is some distance from the everyday life of the ward the patient who is secluded is given an implicit message of expulsion from the community. This can exacerbate his mental state and cause the seclusion to last longer.

The furnishings of the seclusion rooms that have been reported are testimony to the stark reality of the lack of development in the use of seclusion down the years. Redmond (1980) offers the following portrayal: 'A seclusion room in a psychiatric facility is devoid of furnishings except perhaps for a mattress'. From this bareness there are references to a number of factors relating to the patient's comfort. For example, Gibson (1989) mentions that lighting should be controlled from outside the seclusion room, and that heating units should be placed high, out of the reach of patients. The seclusion room decor should be bright and airy, according to Craig, Ray and Hix (1989) and, as time for the patient in seclusion becomes distorted (Barradell, 1985), the patient should have sight of a clock. Depending on the patient's mental state any number of personal possessions should be allowed, up to and including the furnishings, as in ordinary rooms (Wells, 1972).

With modern architectural developments there is a tendency towards the custom building of a suite of rooms, which includes a seclusion room, a restraint room, a bathroom, anteroom and lockers, all incorporated as a small unit within the main ward (Craig, Ray and Hix, 1989).

RESTRAINT

The majority of the articles on seclusion emanate from the USA, and there is considerable overlap between the use of mechanical restraints and the use of seclusion. However, from the fewer references from British sources it would appear that mechanical restraints are used far less frequently, and perhaps in some cases seclusion has supplanted them. The main thrust of the argument for the use of restraints to replace seclusion is the insistence that a staff member must always be in attendance on a person mechanically restrained. It must also be noted that ' . . . locked seclusion and locked wards cannot be considered less restrictive and carry with them the risk that the patient will injure himself while unattended' (Rosen and di Giacomo, 1978).

While restraint with strong suits, straitjackets and posey belts is sometimes used on patients in seclusion, by and large such restraints are used instead of seclusion. If the imagery of a person locked in a seclusion room is found to be unacceptable, then surely a person tied in strong suits and straitjackets is equally unacceptable? What, then, of chemical restraint? The use of seclusion and medication is also suggested to be as restrictive as mechanical restraints, with medication appearing more sinister. As Bursten (1975) suggested, 'when a patient suddenly becomes self-injurious and is given medication, it is often given by injection to control, sedate and chemically restrain him'.

The idea that chemical restraint is more acceptable because it cannot be seen, as a seclusion room or straitjacket can, may be a pointer to understanding why the sight of a fellow human being, held fastened, evokes such negative emotions.

TYPES OF ESTABLISHMENT

On considering a wide range of articles on seclusion from around the world it can be seen that seclusion is used in many different contexts and settings, from institutions such as private voluntary clinics to maximum-security establishments for the dangerous, violent and criminally insane. Clearly, the types of clientele catered for and the policies and practices of the units concerned contribute to the use of seclusion. For example, Wells' (1972) study, in which he reports that 4% of patients on their unit are secluded, is referring to a university medical centre psychiatric floor with a 12-bedded locked area. This teaching unit has a small number of general psychiatric patients with considerable staff input, a multidisciplinary approach, and work along intensive, individualized, care plan lines.

Other studies reporting relatively low seclusion rates include that of Soloff (1978), whose setting was two acute inpatient units of a large military teaching hospital. A private voluntary psychiatric division of a general hospital consisting of six inpatient units was the setting for Mattson and Sacks' (1978) study, which reported that 7.2% of their patients were secluded.

The majority of studies in the literature reviewed relate to general psychiatric patients in either state hospitals (Plutchik *et al.*, 1978; Tardiff, 1981; Philips and Nasr, 1983) or university teaching hospitals (Schwab and Lahmeyer, 1979; Gerlock and Solomons, 1983; Oldham, Russakoff and Prusnofsky, 1983), who all report a wide disparity of seclusion usage, and it would appear that the specific philosophy or function of the unit is a major determinant in its implementation. For example, Binder (1979) reported seclusion rates of 44% when work is within the directive 'Seclusion is to be used whenever a patient is presented to the unit and there is a history of, or threat of, violence or when a prospective patient has been brought in by the police' (Binder, 1979). As many patients have a history of violence, and as the police are often involved in patient admissions, this must clearly be responsible in part for the high seclusion figures reported.

The highest reported seclusion rate located in this review (66%) was in a study by Wadeson and Carpenter (1976) on an NIMH clinical research unit for acute schizophrenic hospitalized patients. However, they argued that 'On this unit, pharmacotherapy was not used during investigative procedures and, in keeping with the unit's treatment philosophy, was used sparingly or not at all during non-investigative periods' (Wadeson and Carpenter, 1976). The result of this philosophy, they suggest, was frequent use of seclusion rooms for severe management problems.

ASSOCIATED FACTORS

In attempts to understand the experience and employment of seclusion some studies have focused upon specific aspects in relation to its use.

Precipitating events

The literature reviewed highlights attempts to establish empirical data on the subfactor of the precipitating events in relation to seclusion initiation. For example, reasons for initiating seclusion have been relatively well reported, although inconclusively, some identifying overt violence as the major determinant for seclusion (Soloff and Turner, 1981; Thompson, 1987), while others have reported no significant difference between actual and threatened violence (Plutchik *et al.*, 1978; Philips and Nasr, 1983; Oldham, Russakoff and Prusnofsky, 1983). There are also some studies that have suggested that it is not violence which is the major determinant for seclusion but behaviour considered to be disruptive to the environment, which is of greater significance (Mattson and Sacks, 1978). They report 34.4% for behaviour disruptive to the environment, with 25.1% for actual assault on others.

However, some authors have reported rather vague reasons for the use of seclusion; for example, Schwab and Lahmeyer (1979) report the major reason for seclusion as being 'destimulation'. This appears to be an all-encompassing word and could be a rationale for almost anything. There is also some disparity in the relatively few studies that report 'dangerous to self' as a reason for seclusion (Plutchik *et al.*, 1978; Thompson, 1987) with a range of 0.5–15% respectively; however, other studies include this criterion for seclusion under the general heading of actual or threatened violence. Baxter, Hale and Hafner (1989) recorded 100% of patients in their study as being secluded for violence, actual or threatened, towards others, themselves or property. Their breakdown figures highlighted a differing pattern between men and women. For example, men who were violent towards staff accounted for 85% of their seclusion figures, whereas male violence towards other patients accounted for 46%; violence towards themselves accounted for 27%, and violence towards property 6%. On the other hand, with women who were violent towards staff they recorded 45%; towards other patients, 29%; towards themselves, 39% and towards property 12% (percentages add up to more than 100, due to more than one reason being given).

Way (1986) recorded 30% of patients secluded in his study as having assaulted a member of staff, with 21% assaulting another patient, 16% demonstrating threatening behaviour, and 16% showing agitated behaviour, with the remainder having a variety of reasons.

Although the precipitating events reported are varied, there appears to be an implicit message within the rationales given for seclusion usage which has echoes of violence and aggression. For example, there appears to be a suggestion that 'destimulation' is required because 'overstimulation' will result in aggression; or that a 'disturbed milieu' will inevitably lead to a 'disturbed' individual becoming violent.

Numbers of patients involved and times of the day

The percentage rates of patients involved in seclusion are wide ranging indeed, from Tardiff's (1981) 1.9% to Wadeson and Carpenter's (1976) 66%. The other studies that report the percentage rates of seclusion use are more or less evenly distributed throughout the range.

These percentage rates should not be viewed in isolation, as there are several factors that may contribute to their production. For example, the general philosophy of the wards and units is a strong factor in determining the use of seclusion. In Wadeson and Carpenter's (1976) study (66%) the unit staff involved did not believe in the use of medication, and therefore the psychotic disturbances were more frequent. This led to an increased use of seclusion, which the unit staff believed to be a much lesser intrusion for the patient than chemical restraint.

In Tardiff's (1981) study based in a state hospital in America, the 1.9% seclusion figure is reflective of the other measures used to control disruptive behaviour. For example, emergency administration of medication was used in 42.8% of cases under study, and 16% received one-to-one observations, with 13% receiving both. The remaining 27.3% was made up of a combination of seclusion, restraints, medication and one-to-one observations and, in some cases, all four at the same time.

The timing of seclusion episodes also shows some variance throughout the literature. For example, Plutchik *et al.* (1978) report 47% during the daytime, 32% in the evening and 21% at night, whereas the figures are almost inverted in Convertino, Pinto and Fiesta's (1980) study, with 15% in the daytime, 41% in the evening and 44% at night. Baxter, Hale and Hafner (1989) reported 19% of seclusion initiations occurring between 0700 and 1100 hours, with 31% between 1100 and 1500 hours. There were 25% between 1500 and 1900 hours, 21% between 1900 and 2300 hours and only 4% during the night. This is a similar pattern to Way's (1986) figures, which show peak periods of seclusion occurring between 0900 and 1000 hours, and between 1200 and

1300 hours, and then falling slowly to reach the lowest period between 0100 and 0600 hours. However, the reasons for these differences may be based on the differing types of establishment in which the studies were undertaken and the differing staffing ratios, both staff/patient and male/female staff, over the 24-hour period.

Staffing ratios

Several authors have suggested that staffing ratios and staff experience affect seclusion rates (Mendel and Green, 1967; Gerlock and Solomons, 1983). However, Schwab and Lahmeyer (1979) found no correlation between age and nursing experience and frequency of seclusion episodes, whereas Morrison and le Roux (1987) concluded that 'The level of experience of the nurse in charge of a ward appears to relate strongly with a tendency to use seclusion'. This must be seen in relation to staffing levels that affect the experience of nurses in charge. As they suggest in their study, 'seclusions were indeed unavoidable because the staffing level was inadequate' (Morrison and le Roux, 1987). However, in a later study Morrison reported that higher rates of seclusion were linked to higher levels of staffing (Morrison, P., 1990).

Kirkpatrick (1989) identified a pattern of seclusions occurring twice as often during shifts which had predominantly male staff, but was unable to produce statistical significance due to the low number of incidents.

There are a number of possible reasons for these disparate results. The general culture of the wards in which seclusion is used may influence its use, especially if the image portrayed is one of toughness and dominance (Morrison, E., 1990a). This is a particular problem in some institutional settings that have a custodial or security function enmeshed with a therapeutic role, and can lead to the reinforcing of seclusion practice as a form of social control. The ramifications are complex and can include such factors as peer-group pressures, subconscious motivations and sadistic tendencies.

However, it may not always be as sinister as this; it may be that increased staffing brings with it increased scrutiny, which may increase stresses and tensions among staff and patients, thus causing seclusion rates to be higher. Unfortunately, reducing staffing levels may also raise tensions, with staff becoming fearful of violent episodes without the facility of sufficiently available support staff, which may encourage the pre-emptive use of seclusion.

Modal durations

Average modal durations of seclusion ranged from 1.25 hours (Oldham, Russakoff and Prusnofsky, 1983) to 25 hours (Wells, 1972), and once again the rationale for this disparity was suggested to be the differing types of establishments, clientele and staffing ratios. Soloff and Turner (1981) reported a mean duration of 10.8 hours in a study of two inpatient units in a university hospital, whereas Plutchik *et al.* (1978) reported a mean duration of 4.1 hours in a municipal hospital; and Binder (1979) quotes an average of 15.7 hours for a crisis intervention unit. There is no statistical significance reported in relation to specific diagnoses or precipitating factors and the duration of seclusion. This raises serious issues, as Soloff (1987) states: 'From a purely legal perspective the wide disparity in seclusion times and the independence of duration from precipitating behaviour and diagnosis braves the unpleasant question of arbitrariness in determining duration: a needlessly prolonged seclusion is a punitive sanction'.

In the contrasting durations of seclusion outlined, the relationship between diagnosis and duration would be difficult to establish, as the categorization of, say, schizophrenia would not take into account the individual nature of each and every schizophrenic involved. However, Soloff (1987) is justifiably concerned, as there may indeed be a relationship between the length of a seclusion and the precipitating behaviour, especially if that behaviour involved assaults on staff.

PATIENT CHARACTERISTICS

The personal characteristics of the patients involved in seclusion episodes have been studied, but with little real consensus as regards the results.

Diagnostic categories

Seclusion of patients in relation to diagnostic categories is more consistent in the literature reviewed, as all but one study (Campbell, Shepard and Falconer, 1982) reported patients with psychotic diagnoses showing an increase in seclusion rates of approximately 3:1 over patients with non-psychotic diagnoses. However, the breakdown of the psychotic grouping highlighted some differences in seclusion rates. In reporting for schizophrenia Binder (1979) shows 36%, with Oldham, Russakoff and Prusnofsky (1983) reporting 41% and Soloff and Turner (1981) similar figures of 42% while Plutchik *et al.* (1978) record the highest rate at 64%.

Baxter, Hale and Hafner (1989) reported that 50% of patients in their study were diagnosed as suffering from schizophrenia or being schizoaffective, with affective disorders 24%, psychopathic disorders 19% and alcoholic hallucinosis 6%.

Way and Banks (1990), in a study of 23 state hospitals in America, produced a table which showed that 54.2% of patients who were secluded during their study were diagnosed as suffering from schizophrenia, with personality disorders at 15.1%, the mentally retarded 12.3%, alcohol and drug-related 8.9%, bipolar disorders 6.4% and the remaining 3.1% with variable diagnoses.

Although there appears to be a general agreement regarding the diagnostic categories and the relationship to seclusion usage, when the categories are subdivided the relationships become somewhat more tenuous. Perhaps more importantly, patients are secluded because of what they do and, it is hoped, not because of what they are. It is interesting to observe that psychotics are secluded more often than non-psychotics, but it does beg the question, why?

Age ranges

The average ages of patients secluded range from 26 years (Oldham, Russakoff and Prusnofsky, 1983) to 36 years (Thompson, 1986), with a general consensus that there is a greater rate of seclusions in the younger patients, diminishing steadily with age. Way and Banks (1990) reported, that patients under the age of 26 years were four times as likely to be secluded than a patient who was over 35 years of age.

With the majority of studies that have reported for age ranges indicating that the younger patient is more likely to be secluded, there is a tendency to lay the blame for this on the impetuosity of youth. It may, however, be more complicated than this, with such traits as the antiauthoritarian and confrontational tendencies of the young adult generally forming the individual's personality. There is no reason to suggest that merely because a person becomes mentally ill the sociocultural components of their character become tempered; indeed, it may be that they become exaggerated.

Gender

Way and Banks (1990) found that within certain age bandings females were significantly more likely to be secluded than males. Soloff and Turner (1981) reported that there was no significant difference between genders for both secluded and non-secluded patients in their study.

HMSO (1980) observed, in the hospital that they were currently investigating, that ' . . . on any one day between 7% and 9% of the female population were likely to be secluded, compared with under 1% of the men' (HMSO, 1980). Clearly, these figures and studies which are at variance confound the issue further. Seclusion and gender requires a much closer examination, particularly in relation to such factors as self-harming behaviours, histories of sexual abuse, and the male–female power/dominance relationship.

Ethnicity

Ethnicity is another important area within the seclusion debate, but is also under-represented in the literature. Flaherty and Meagher (1980) attempted to measure racial bias in an inpatient treatment centre, with the use of seclusion as one of the many variables under investigation. They reported that seclusion and restraints were used for blacks on 78% of the days of hospitalization, and for whites on 46%, and they concluded that there was some evidence of racial bias on their unit.

Carpenter *et al.* (1988b) studied the ethnic differences in seclusion and restraints in the New York State mental hospital system. Their breakdown was whites 59.8%, blacks 31.3% and Hispanics

8.9%. Having analysed their data with a battery of statistical tests they concluded: 'These findings suggest that systematic bias in confinement of racial groups does not exist in New York State psychiatric hospitals, although this does not rule out the possibility that some other type of bias may exist' (Carpenter *et al.*, 1988b).

Lawson, Yesavage and Werner (1984), in a similar study, had reported that 'Item analysis revealed that Whites made more violent threats, committed more violent acts against self, and were more likely to be secluded or restrained'.

These three examples show quite clearly that there are wide variations in the published literature regarding the role of ethnicity and seclusion use. It is without doubt a clear area for further research.

Legal status

From a study set in a general hospital in America, Ramchandani, Akhtar and Helfrich (1981) found, perhaps not too surprisingly, that involuntary patients were secluded more often than those of voluntary status. They also noted that the involuntary patient was perceived differently by both staff and voluntary patients, who viewed them as 'disturbed, upset and angry'. These results were supported by Oldham, Russakoff and Prusnofsky (1983), who also found that involuntary patients in their study were more often secluded than voluntary patients.

A more complex study by Soloff and Turner (1981) did not support Ramchandani's (1981) study, as the former reported that 63% of '... patients were on voluntary status prior to their first seclusion and only 37% under commitment'. However, two things should be observed in these findings. The first is that involuntary status was closely associated with the diagnosis of psychosis and the second is that the pattern reversed itself for schizophrenic patients, who accounted for 64% of seclusions while on involuntary status.

Philips and Nasr (1983) reported that they found no significant difference between voluntary and involuntary patients in their study.

Where it may be thought that compulsorily detained patients would be generally thought to be more dangerous, it might be expected that they would be secluded more often. However, from the foregoing studies the issue is clearly much more complicated than this, and it is hoped that the issue will receive due investigation in future research projects.

Length of stay

Seclusion use in relation to length of stay has also been studied, but by no means in depth, with, once again, disparate results reported. Tardiff (1981) produced the figure of 70.7% of seclusion use ' . . . in those patients who had spent 10 or more years in the hospital'. This was supported by Soloff and Turner (1981), who also found that their ' . . . secluded sample tended towards a longer hospital stay'. This was countered by Oldham, Russakoff and Prusnofsky (1983), who found no significant differences between secluded and non-secluded groups of patients in relation to length of stay.

In a more recent study (Way and Banks, 1990), the above results were reversed and they reported that ' . . . patients who were secluded or restrained had significantly shorter lengths of hospitalisation than those who were not'. They also pointed out that patients with longer lengths of stay had a greater probability of being secluded, but added that this effect varied due to interactions with other variables, a point which is not lost in respect of the abundance of variables in the seclusion research.

OTHER FACTORS

Other, more unusual, factors associated with use of seclusion have been studied by Gerlock and Solomons (1983), who investigated variations in cyclic phenomena (earth and biological cycles), and found that more seclusions occurred during winter and spring, and most during April and January. However, they found no significant difference between lunar phases, little variation throughout the week and no relationship between seclusion and precipitation, barometric pressure readings and barometric pressure changes. They had no data on menstrual or circadian cycles, and no significant differences were apparent between secluded and control group for biorhythms, horoscopes or birth signs.

PATIENTS' RESPONSES

It is interesting to note, in the relatively few studies that address the issue of the patients' responses to seclusion, that 'When they represented their affect in drawings it was always negative. This is in contrast to reports in debriefing interviews at discharge and follow-ups where various ideas and feelings about seclusion are described, by no means all were negative' (Wadeson and Carpenter, 1976). In another study there were a number of responses from patients as to their feelings while in seclusion. Some thought predominantly about their release, while others focused on the injustice of their seclusion. Some concentrated on the passage of time and others described feelings of intense anger, depression or abandonment. When asked in retrospect whether seclusion had been helpful to them, 41% felt it had had a calming effect on them, but an equal number said it had not helped them in any way. The patients' perspective on seclusion is developed more fully in Chapter 11.

ATTITUDES TO SECLUSION

The literature reviewed highlighted both negative and positive attitudes from both staff and patients, but usually with discrepancies between the two. For example, in a study of 32 nurses and 30 patients who had been involved in seclusion, they were asked to state the facts of their seclusion experience, their beliefs about its use and their feelings concerning change. The study concluded: ' . . . there existed a discrepancy between what nursing staff state their attitude toward seclusion and the secluded patient was, and what is exhibited or implied through their behaviour' (Heyman, 1987).

When staff are asked about their attitude to seclusion as a safe and effective therapeutic tool, they tend to report positively and unambiguously in support (Kilgalen, 1977; Plutchik et al., 1978; Soloff and Turner, 1981; Soliday, 1985). However, this has to be contrasted with some considerable disquiet reported by staff in other studies regarding seclusion usage (Fitzgerald and Long, 1973; Strutt et al., 1980; Convertino, Pinto and Fiesta, 1980; Campbell, Shepard and Falconer, 1982).

In Plutchik et al.'s (1978) study of staff and patients' attitudes towards seclusion it was found that staff satisfaction was high, with seclusion helping the ward run smoothly and helping the patient gain stability, but regret that alternatives were unavailable.

Although the relatively few studies carried out on staff and patients' attitudes to seclusion do not represent a thorough examination, it is suggested that certain trends are emerging: first, that patients generally regard seclusion as negative, despite some believing it to be necessary; and secondly that staff generally regard it as positive, despite some disquiet over its use (Hodgkinson, 1985).

The attitude to seclusion is often reported as a necessary evil with regard to the lack of options, and 'Perhaps the principal reason for the use of seclusion is the unsatisfactory nature of the alternatives' (Angold, 1989).

CONCLUSION

It is often difficult to appreciate the abundance of factors that contribute to the use of seclusion, and indeed the policy formulation, the monitoring systems and the research studies initiated to unravel some of its complexities. From the foregoing extensive, but perhaps not exhaustive, literature review it is apparent that over the past two decades the increased public scrutiny caused by litigation in the courts has focused attention on the issue. Perhaps it would be somewhat cynical to suggest that without this publicity professional motivation to review the practice would have remained to a large extent dormant. However, whatever the cause of the increased interest, the point is that seclusion is now investigated more closely than ever before, and is likely to continue to be so for some considerable time to come.

The legal ramifications of direct liability under the law, and from internal and public inquiries, are now extensive, and without doubt affect the way seclusion is practised. It is this interface between law and practice that brings the issue of seclusion to a functional consideration. Seclusion is often used as a crisis intervention for the extremes of disturbed behaviours and, as such, is usually activated at the onset of assaultative action, or immediately prior to it, as a preventative measure. Assessing the prodromal signs and symptoms in relation to outbursts of assault is always difficult, in that, if staff wait too long to intervene then they themselves, or others, may get hurt, and if they intervene too early they are often accused of overreacting. The legal considerations do pressurize the professional practice of secluding patients, in compelling staff to wait until there is an absolute necessity to do so. However, the practical issue in the interim, when other interventions are being attempted, is the consequence of possible failure of these interventions, with the end result likely to be injuries sustained.

When all else fails and the patient is actually in the throes of combat, there is quite clearly an urgency, indeed a duty, to intervene, be that seclusion or restraint. We feel there is no case for allowing the freedom of bodily movement when that movement is an attack on another person. The difficulty for staff is in the timing of the intervention, which cannot be completely right on all occasions. When the political, professional, practical, personal and legal factors are constantly being brought to bear on any decision, as they must, then sometimes the decisions turn out to be the wrong ones.

It is little wonder, therefore, that within the literature on seclusion, including the inquiry reports and the court transcripts, the use of seclusion is referred to sometimes positively, frequently neutrally and often negatively. With this in mind a theoretical framework can be established which involves the use of seclusion as a therapeutic intervention, as a means of containment or as a form of punishment.

4

Seclusion as therapy, containment or punishment

Tom Mason

The theory relating to seclusion is slowly evolving, but since the pioneering works of Gutheil (1978), who made some central observations on the theoretical base for seclusion, and Plutchik *et al.* (1978) who developed a rationale for the seclusion process, there has been little attention paid to the theoretical constructs. This is not to say that great efforts have not been made to study the factors associated with seclusion use: indeed, quite the contrary, as the literature review clearly shows. However, the central tenets of the seclusion theory, outlined in the above studies in 1978, have remained relatively unaltered, although it is fair to say that they have been drawn together on numerous occasions (Hodgkinson, 1985; Soloff, Gutheil and Wexlet, 1985; Angold, 1989) and only marginally developed recently (Roper *et al.*, 1985; Mason 1993a).

In this chapter we intend to draw together the major theoretical constructs of seclusion, and to identify an overall framework on which to base future debate. From the literature reviews undertaken the seclusion theory may be summarized as being underpinned by one of three basic rationales. First, seclusion is seen as a therapeutic intervention (T); secondly, it may be a means of containment (C); and thirdly, it may be a form of punishment (P). Although, as will be seen, and as we readily accept, there is often a great deal of overlap within the 'TCP' structure which accounts for the complexity and contentiousness of the seclusion issue.

Each central tenet of the 'TCP' framework will be examined,

from both positive and negative aspects, which may be located on what may be called a benevolent–malevolent (B–M) scale (Mason, 1993a) (Figure 4.1).

Within this framework we can locate the theoretical components that constitute the general theory of seclusion.

SECLUSION AS A THERAPEUTIC INTERVENTION (T)

Seclusion as a benevolent therapeutic intervention is put forward in the literature as an appropriate mode of treatment based on sound curative principles. Although it is sometimes not clear whether the argument is that the seclusion room *per se* is inherently therapeutic, it is certainly the case that the 'act' of putting someone into seclusion is stated to be therapeutically beneficial. It has been argued that seclusion is a therapeutic method of treating severely ill patients with an array of psychiatric disorders. However, it has also been reported that it is of

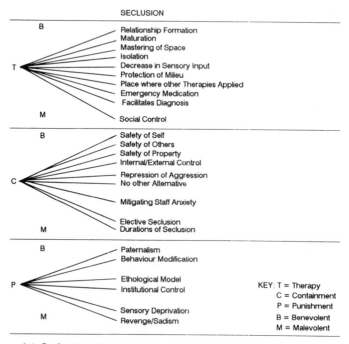

Figure 4.1 Seclusion theory constructs in relation to a benevolent–malevolent scale

particular benefit with manic and depressed patients, and that seclusion has served '. . . to help build sound psychotherapeutic relationships . . . ' (Fitzgerald and Long, 1973). It would appear that these authors suggest that the process of intervention, in the form of seclusion, reassures the patient by indicating that no matter what the depth of their disturbance, they will receive a therapeutic intervention from the nursing staff.

The establishment of therapeutic relationships was also emphasized by Schwab and Lahmeyer (1979), who argued strongly in favour of much reduced medication despite higher rates of seclusion, as they felt that the former was not in the best interests of patients.

Seclusion as a therapeutic intervention also includes its use in approaching aggressive behaviour from a psychodynamic perspective, according to Grigson (1984). This means using seclusion as a mechanism for addressing the patient's maturational needs, which involves the patient's own self-assessment in relation to development strategies. Within this approach it is argued that '. . . we have successfully begun to deal with the interferences in maturation that cause these patients to maintain the same impulsive and destructive behavioural patterns for most of their lives . . . ' (Grigson, 1984). Although not totally clear, it is assumed that the patient gains some therapeutic insights from the seclusion process which, notwithstanding Grigson's stated psychodynamic approach, may in real terms be behaviouralistic in nature.

The author coming perhaps closest to seclusion *per se* as a therapeutic intervention mentioned it only in passing, and as a corollary of it, and that was Gutheil (1978) with the notion of 'mastery of space'. This theoretical concept involves the patient's access to areas of the ward being restricted, at first, so that they establish the ability to cope with the increasing encounters and surprises that the ward environment holds. Once familiar and capable of interacting appropriately with a level of free access, then more areas are opened up to them for additional possibilities, and so on, until they become accomplished on the entire ward, then the hospital, and ultimately society. The seclusion room is the smallest space on the graduated system, and represents for the patient an area that can be mastered, holds few surprises and can be seen in its entirety without hidden threats. Gutheil (1978) called it 'the zero point'.

Isolation

The principle of isolation addresses the issue of the patient's vulnerability to ' . . . a variety of forms of pathological intensity in relationships . . . ' (Gutheil, 1978), the argument being that relationships, particularly when they are prone to serious misinterpretations, become problematic for the patient who has no means of escaping this intensity, and seclusion is a means of relief from this torment (Plutchik *et al.*, 1978).

The isolation postulate is founded on the notion of decreasing the emotional input that it is believed the patient is vulnerable to, particularly the paranoid patient. Relationships between staff and patients can become demanding and 'at times these may be open to misinterpretation . . . or the demand from staff for patients to assume greater responsibility, or insight into their feelings and actions may become intolerable and be rejected. A period in the seclusion room restricts the number and nature of such demands on the patient' (Hodgkinson, 1985). Here it is suggested that the demands of therapeutic activity can become a burden on the patient, who needs time away from the stress. However, it must surely be arguable whether seclusion is the appropriate place for such respite.

Not only is the application of therapeutic interventions suggested to cause stress within patients, particularly psychotics, but environmental aspects of the unit itself can also overload the patient, and ' . . . the inability to tolerate stimuli from the environment is manifested by increasing levels of agitation and seclusion. The reduction of sensory stimulation . . . achieved with seclusion, can help the patient to tolerate incoming stimuli' (McCoy and Garritson, 1983).

Decrease in sensory input

Although related to the isolation principle this concept involves sensory input along all modalities of perception. This need for 'destimulation' is well reported in the literature (Fitzgerald and Long, 1973; Kilgalen, 1977; Schwab and Lahmeyer, 1979) and is based on the widely held belief that certain patients suffer because of excessive internal mental activity, which is stimulated by an overloading of external stimuli. There is considerable support for the use of seclusion as a method of decreasing this input.

Rosen and di Giacomo (1978) identified four indicators for the use of physical restraints in the effort to reduce sensory stimuli: first, violent behaviour which cannot be adequately controlled by other techniques; secondly, the presence of marked agitation, thought disorder or severe confusion when the patient's physical condition limits the use of psychotropic medication; thirdly, hyperactivity, insomnia, decreased food and fluid intake, and grossly impaired judgement, particularly when accompanied by regressed socially unacceptable behaviour; and fourthly, when it is requested by the patient. However, the appropriateness of secluding a patient (let alone using physical restraints) who is deemed to be severely confused or has problems with eating or sleeping is highly questionable and, as McCoy and Garritson (1983) suggest, 'depends on whether those problems necessitate external controls via seclusion rather than offering a low-stimulus environment'.

At a middle point on the B–M scale in relation to seclusion as a therapeutic intervention is the notion that the seclusion room itself is not the therapy but merely the place in which therapies can be applied. The majority of writers on seclusion argue that contact with the patient during this time is both crucial and central in establishing therapeutic links. Whether it be for assessment of the patient's mental state or for an educative approach in teaching the patient alternative behavioural strategies, contact time is always emphasized as being of vital importance. This indicates that something additional to seclusion is manifestly important for the progress of the patient. Rather than isolation, the secluded patient ' . . . requires much intensive treatment and observation' (McCoy and Garritson, 1983). This brings seclusion within the special care framework and reinforces the idea that it is a time in which other nursing interventions are applied, rather than waiting and hoping that something will change within the patient.

The use of seclusion is closely linked to the administration of emergency medication, either at the time of the incident leading to its implementation or shortly afterwards. This is clearly an intervention above and beyond the use of seclusion as a therapeutic approach and, with the use of sedating drugs, seclusion becomes an area of intensified nursing.

It has been argued that seclusion has therapeutic benefits for the patient, in that the control of certain behaviours aids early diagnosis and thus facilitates prompt psychiatric interventions (Fitzgerald and Long, 1973). The supporting rationale for this approach is that severely disturbed individuals who may be out of control on the ward, running rampant, shouting incoherently, engaging in destructive behaviour, and unable or unwilling to sit and talk, are better confined to a distinct area, i.e. seclusion. This places the patient in one small area, so that nursing staff can focus their attention, identify more specific patterns of behaviour and are more likely to be able to communicate with the patient. It is suggested that, in many cases, once a diagnosis has been identified seclusion is no longer deemed the appropriate intervention and is therefore terminated. Fitzgerald and Long (1973) offer a case scenario of an overactive and destructive lady being admitted in an acute frenzy who may have received a diagnosis of mania, established from a distance. However, once placed in seclusion it became apparent to the staff that acute schizophrenia was the more appropriate diagnosis. Seclusion was terminated and she received the appropriate care from those most experienced in treating this illness. It is reported that she made a swift and full recovery.

We would argue that this rationale for seclusion can be located towards the neutral point on the therapeutic B–M scale, because seclusion is not perceived as a specific therapeutic intervention but as a form of behaviourial control to aid diagnosis. It may be argued that this rationale may be better placed within the containment principle. However, as the rationale is underpinned by the ultimate application of a treatment modality we feel it is more appropriately situated within the therapeutic framework; but, as pointed out earlier, we accept a great deal of overlap.

Also, within the more neutral mode of the B–M therapeutic scale is the protection of the milieu as a rationale for the seclusion. This is, once again, placed within the therapeutic framework as the ultimate intention is that the milieu, as a treatment, be safeguarded and allowed to continue to act as a treatment, at least for all the other patients that are not secluded. However, it must be remembered that the milieu as a treatment modality is somewhat tenuous; that the utilitarian position has been heavily criticized; and that the slippage of the underlying rationale towards containment and/or punishment can be considerable. However, it has been, and still is, offered in the literature as a contribution towards an understanding of the seclusion theory.

The theory is that seclusion can protect the therapeutic activity of the ward environment, and that this enhances the mental welfare of the remaining non-secluded patients. It is also suggested that, rather than the secluded patient suffering for the greater benefit of the majority, seclusion intervenes by preventing a deterioration in that patient's mental state.

The application of a therapeutic technique at a malevolent level may at first be difficult to accept. (By acceptance we mean acceptance of the event occurring and not acceptance of the propriety of the act.) We would also make a distinction between conscious maleficent punishment and a subconscious, or unknown, malevolent therapy. The former will be examined later; the latter is dealt with here, within the therapeutic framework, as to all intents and purposes the staff involved are either ignorant of the malevolence within the intervention or are bigoted in their denial of its existence; or are dismissive of it and resort to the dogma of traditional medical and nursing ideology for support. If there is any difficulty in appreciating that doctors and nurses can, sometimes unknowingly, develop malevolent practices, one needs only to turn to the Holocaust, where their role is increasingly being examined following almost 40 years of silence on the topic. It is easy to assume that those doctors and nurses who took part in the early 'euthanasias' and the developing programmes of assessment of 'fitness to life' were both evil and culpable, and their actions indefensible. However, at the Nuremberg trials the testimonies of those involved showed that they not only vigorously defended their actions, but also firmly believed that what they did was correct and appropriate, given the historical development of the German culture. It is clear from the transcripts that they believed in the correctness of their actions as much as the prosecutors believed in their impropriety. This is an example of how dogma and bigotry, on all sides, can so easily lead to narrowness of thought and entrenched positions being taken up without any analysis or understanding of the alternative viewpoints: a condition very reminiscent of the seclusion debate.

The antipsychiatry lobby have argued that the whole notion of mental illness is a myth (Szasz, 1962) and that supposed psychiatric interventions are, at best, forms of social control, and at worst, external signs of a degenerating society. It is suggested that the social construction of what is termed madness is part of the wider dissolution of relationships between individuals, and that the forced application of treatment in these areas represents a wider social problem. Within this theoretical framework psychiatry is seen as an interference in a person's right to behaviours which are non-harmful to others. These behaviours may lead to the label 'madness' but, Szasz would ask, whose madness is it?

Another well known antipsychiatrist who lobbied hard for the patients' rights to be themselves was R.D. Laing. He argued that psychiatry, in its current form, was little more than a punitive controlling mechanism: 'it is a ceremonial of control, control of mind, body and conduct, and always, whatever else, control for the sake of sheer control, of more control, of perfect, complete control' (Laing, 1982).

Therapy as a malevolent intervention was also advanced by Michel Foucault, particularly the treatment of the mentally ill. Foucault suggested that the power of medicine to identify illness, through technological and classificatory systems, forced those so identified on a 'journey' from a condition of abnormality to a state of normality (Foucault, 1967). A 'journey', Foucault argued, with no point of disembarkation for many, as the state of normality was unobtainable for them. The seclusion of mentally ill patients for reasons of therapy can be seen as part and parcel of this forced 'journey' from illness to 'wellness'. Some patients, particularly the mentally impaired and the chronic mentally ill, will remain on this journey forever.

SECLUSION AS A MEANS OF CONTAINMENT (C)

Eliminating both the therapeutic and punitive rationales for the use of seclusion leaves us with the containment principle. Containment is the end result of perhaps many failed alternative interventions, and it is used when the patient is in the act of assault, or when it is considered that assault is imminent. The theoretical underpinnings to the containment principle can also range from benevolence through to malevolence, with what may be termed areas of neutrality in between.

Perhaps the starting point, at the benevolent end of the scale, is that the containment principle is based on the ' . . . restriction of a patient's movement to a place that is safe from both self-injury and the possibly damaging consequences of injury to others' (Gutheil, 1978). A third factor in the safety of self and others criterion can be identified in the literature, and that is the protection of property (Gutheil, 1978; Tardiff, 1984).

The seclusion of patients for their own safety has been theorized on several levels. First, that the patient who is prone to self-injury often finds the containment of their destructive behaviours by seclusion reassuring, and this is a fundamental need of the patient (Mattson and Sacks, 1978). The seclusion room is a containing mechanism while an intensive programme is organized. Clearly, it is in the patient's best interests not to harm himself, as this can only cause more pain and injury. Seclusion and other methods are offered as an appropriate strategy for dealing with such cases. Secondly, it is suggested that seclusion may be used not only for patients who self-injure, but also for those who emit behaviours while 'ill' which, when 'well', they would be highly ashamed of or embarrassed about. The protection of the patient's dignity and feelings of guilt by using seclusion, if alternatives fail, is considered appropriate in some cases (Kilgalen, 1977).

Seclusion for the protection of others is also firmly rooted in the benevolent containment principle, in that other patients and staff have a right not to be attacked and sustain injuries. Despite some suggestions that, with alternative techniques, violent outbreaks on the ward can be reduced to a minimum, aggression and assaults do still occur. It is argued that the containment of such assaultative behaviours by the use of seclusion is in the attacker's best interest, on two counts. First, the assaulted patient may take some form of retaliatory physical action, which in some cases may be extreme and has certainly been known to result in murder. Secondly, the assaulted person may have recourse to the law, which may lead to severe penalties for the attacker. Prompt intervention in an attack, or even a pre-emptive intervention by using seclusion to prevent a situation deteriorating, can thus be seen as benevolent containment.

Seclusion has also been justified for those patients who may be at serious risk of destroying property (Gutheil *et al.*, 1984). Clearly, it is not in the patient's interest to destroy large amounts of property, no matter who it belongs to, on the grounds that he may have to replace the equipment, reimburse others or pay hospital bills for damage caused. Once again the destructive patient may be retaliated against or subjected to litigation, or possibly face criminal proceedings, for example in the case of arson. Despite the Mental Health Act Code of Practice (HMSO,

1990) stating that seclusion should not be used because '... equipment is being damaged', it could be argued that there are occasions when all other interventions have failed, when the use of seclusion is appropriate, not for therapeutic reasons, nor for punitive ones, but merely to contain the situation, in the patient's own best interests.

The containment of a person in seclusion as a form of external control in the hope that their own internal control will regain equilibrium is well documented (Kilgalen, 1977; Gutheil, 1978; Redmond, 1980). It is argued that when expectations are known and the consequences of an action are experienced, there is an opportunity for the growth and development of ego strengths. Gentilin (1987) argued that 'a room that is reassuringly familiar can be a safe place that allows this process to happen', and suggests that particularly irresponsible behaviour should be treated in this manner. This application of an external control to maintain a person's internal control is perhaps similar to the external structure of the law, for example, enforcing behaviourial controls on at least some members of society. The external/ internal control theory is based on the idea of the repression of aggression, which is very much a fundamental principle in human development (Binder, 1979; Ramchandani, Akhtar and Helfrich, 1981).

Moving more closely towards the neutral position on the containment B–M scale, it is suggested that seclusion is the safest option for all concerned when a person becomes combatant. Although it may appear that this principle is a surrender to the lack of alternative interventions, it is firmly rooted at a practical level. Clearly, when a person is in the throes of assault something has to be done to stop them. Redmond (1980) summed up the containment ethos as 'seclusion on this unit is not used as punishment or coercion, nor is there any attempt to justify use of seclusion for therapeutic purposes'. This must surely have been a pioneering statement at that time.

Another rationale for seclusion as containment is offered by Fitzgerald and Long (1973), who claim it is justified for allaying staff anxiety, and they illustrate this reasoning with a case history. They report a manic woman about to be admitted on to an already disturbed ward, which was causing the nursing staff a great deal of concern. It was agreed that she would be admitted straight into seclusion, to mitigate staff anxiety and provide them with the opportunity to develop an operational plan that would take into consideration all the circumstances regarding her case. This, we would suggest, fits the neutral containment position, with perhaps a slight leaning towards the malevolent pole, as the major gain from the seclusion is the reduction in staff anxiety rather than the application of something for the patient's benefit. Clearly no punishment is intended, and the therapeutic activity does not involve the seclusion itself: the overriding reason for the use of seclusion is containment.

Malevolent containment quite clearly overlaps considerably with the notion of malevolent punishment. However, the narrow distinction we would make between the two is in terms of the motivation for initiating the seclusion. In the malevolent punishment we see the rationale for secluding the patient as punitively based, whereas at the malevolent containment pole there has been no punitive intention. Seclusion was initiated for containment purposes only, but the malevolence comes in when it is maintained for longer than necessary.

Towards this pole of the containment B–M scale there are a number of rationales, but only two will be focused upon here as it is the theory that underscores the reasoning which is central to the understanding of seclusion use. The first is elective seclusion, which is a particular problem in relation to self-injurious behaviours or threats of self-injury, particularly with those patients who will threaten to harm themselves if they are not put into seclusion. If diversion, dissuasion and alternatives fail, then nursing staff feel pressurized to seclude the patient, not only because they do not wish the patient to injure themselves but also because of the fear of charges of negligence in the event of an actual injury being sustained. The malevolence arises on two levels: first, once a patient elects to go into seclusion the termination is at the will of others; otherwise it is not, by definition, seclusion. This can lead to the duration of seclusion being extended beyond the point that the patient wishes, in order to redress the loss of control felt at having to succumb to the patient's wishes in the first place; the patient's wishes to come out of seclusion are thereby overridden. The second level of malevolence arises with a growing body of evidence in the literature regarding elective seclusion as a form of self-abuse. The staff operating such seclusions are a party to this abuse, although it is fair to say that they may be unaware of this and are often unwilling participants (Burrow 1992; Mason, 1992).

Another example of malevolent containment involves the duration of the seclusion in relation to the reason for its necessity. It is well reported that the duration of seclusion is arbitrary and generally at the whim of the nursing staff (Plutchik *et al.*, 1978; Hodgkinson, 1985; Angold, 1989). However, there is an implicit suggestion that if a member of staff was assaulted, for example, the duration of seclusion would be longer than if another patient had been the recipient of the same type of assault.

SECLUSION AS A FORM OF PUNISHMENT (P)

Seclusion as a form of punishment is generally avoided in the literature on seclusion, presumably due to the strong emotive feelings that are engendered by the notion of punishment and the caring role. Although there are many comments in policy documents and research literature that dismiss any role for punishment in relation to the use of seclusion, these do not eradicate the very fundamental function that punishment plays in human activity. Seclusion as a form of punishment, like therapy and containment, can be located along the B–M scale.

Any parent knows only too well the need for benevolent punishment to control a growing child's behaviour. Whether this means sending children to bed early or withdrawing their pocket money, one would like to think that the punishment was paternalistic and rooted in a genuine caring and compassionate motivation. However, as many child abuse cases inform us, this is not always so. There have been attempts to unravel this perplexing concept of punishment by locating it in terms of a power–authority relationship. Berlin (1975) describes the use of authority and power in a positive light to promote a learning environment (seclusion), and Keith (1984) suggests that some individuals require immediate aversive stimuli (isolation) for them to be able to develop their internal controls. Despite these valid, if somewhat academic, points it appears that the honesty of one's motives for the use of power/authority/punishment is the central issue in carrying out the act, and it must surely be the recipient's perception of the effect of its enactment that features most large for them.

Behaviouralist science deals with the applied experimental

analysis of human behaviour. The conceptual basis that under-
pins behaviour modification forms what is known as modern
learning theory. The main issues in the role of behaviour modification can be summarized into three types of control. First, the
control which is applied without the patient's consent; secondly, control which is directed at the patient's environment to
cause a change in his or her behaviour; and thirdly, the control
the patient manages as a self-monitoring system. The first two
types of control can relate to the seclusion debate, and the argument is based on the ethical implications of the reward and
punishment of human behaviours (Bandura, 1969). It is well
understood that reward and punishment are prominent aspects
in human social activity, but when they become part and parcel
of institutional 'treatment', moral questions abound concerning
the propriety of such approaches. Whether punishment should
be used to alter human behaviour is certainly a very emotive
topic which does not fit well with many practitioners' conceptual
caring framework. However, some scientists have argued that
'recent research . . . indicated that the scientific premises offered
by psychologists for the rejection of punishment are not tenable.
Rather, punishment can be a very useful tool for effecting
behaviour change' (Lovaas *et al.*, 1974).

Towards the neutral point of the B–M scale in relation to
punishment we can situate the ethological model. According
to Plutchik *et al.* (1978): 'In a naturalistic setting in order for a
conglomerate of individuals to be considered a group, there are
a number of requirements that must be met', and they suggest
six fundamental requisites. First, rules of interaction must be
both understood and accepted by the members; secondly, the
rules and (some) members must remain stable over an extended
period of time; thirdly, there must exist a power hierarchy of
domination or authority which will increase the group stability;
fourthly, to ensure adherence to the rules there must be a set of
reinforcements; fifthly, sanctions must be available to the group
in the case of rule breakers; and finally, the group must have an
identified territory of its own.

In terms of the psychiatric ward the above conditions are met
and seclusion is seen as a sanction against rule breakers. There
are several forms of sanction within the ethological model: expulsion, isolation, re-education and execution. Expulsion is not generally used on psychiatric wards, although moving the patient

to higher-dependency areas is a type of expulsion. Execution is not an option, and therefore isolation and re-education are most often used: re-education in the form of treatment, and isolation as seclusion.

The effectiveness of seclusion as a sanction, it is argued, ' . . . is by the fact that the great majority of those group members who break the rules and get secluded do not break the rules again. For the very few who do, it takes some time before they break enough rules to justify their being secluded again' (Plutchik *et al.*, 1978).

Also within the neutral area we can mention the role of punishment in the wider society. No matter how it is dressed up, in terms of rehabilitation or re-education, the fundamental role of punishment is to control behaviour. We are all familiar with the social system of the law, the police, the court and the sentence. The Armed Forces have their Queen's Regulations, prisons have their prison rules, schools have their sanctions and Health Authorities have their disciplinary procedures. Any institution needs measures to control the behaviour of its members, both members who are considered normal (in a state of wellness) and those categorized as abnormal (in a state of illness). The American Psychiatric Association (APA) task force on seclusion and restraint reported that 'it may not be *per se* impermissible to punish mental patients, so long as they are punished for rule-breaking behaviour and not for their status of being mentally ill' (American Psychiatric Association, 1984). However, they went on to argue that if such a system of sanctions were to be applied institutionally then it might become fraught with danger. There would have to be mechanisms established for hearing cases, appeals, proscribed behaviours and appropriate sanctions, of which seclusion must not be one. The task force report that ' . . . the punitive use of seclusion and restraints, while conceptually possible, bristles with clinical, legal, ethical, and policy difficulties and should not ordinarily be resorted to' (APA, 1984). The APA are justifiably concerned, as the slide towards the malevolent pole of the punishment scale is easily achieved.

Seclusion room litigation, as outlined in the Boston State case (see Chapter 5), has given rise (among other things) to a questioning of the moral propriety of its use. There is a suggestion that 'Isolation under the name of 'seclusion' has long been used in mental hospitals as a form of 'treatment' . . . since such isolation tends to promote fantasy regression and bodily illusions in normal subjects, it would seem to be contra-indicated for psychotic patients . . . sensory deprivation experiments support the growing feeling in modern psychiatry that seclusion is harmful to mental patients' (Freedman and Greenblatt, 1960). Although there is little argument that sensory deprivation is harmful to non-psychotics, there remains a degree of controversy over its effects on some psychotic groups and, while suggesting that identifying diagnostic categories which benefit most from seclusion may appear an appropriate proposition, it is probably safer to suggest that it is the individual characteristics of the patient's psychopathology prior to the onset of illness and during the active phase that relate directly to the benefits or otherwise of sensory deprivation. This is supported by the view that 'experimental research demonstrates that individual response to sensory deprivation is remarkably variable; there would be grave risk in assuming that all psychiatric patients – or even the more limited category of actively psychotic patients – would react similarly to psychiatric seclusion' (Grassian and Friedman, 1986).

In sensory deprivation studies on psychiatric patients some authors conclude that, as certain psychotics deteriorate in seclusion, its use is inadmissible on the grounds that there is no means of accurately identifying beforehand who will benefit (Freedman and Greenblatt, 1960; Barton, 1962). However, others have argued along heuristic lines, considering that legal safeguards and constant clinical judgements ensure that the provision of seclusion is a useful treatment modality (Harris, 1957; Grassian and Friedman, 1986).

Further towards the malevolent end of the scale, we can understand the role of revenge in the use of seclusion.

Whaley and Ramirez (1980) reported that in a questionnaire study of mental health professionals 30% admitted the belief that seclusion was used as a punishment. Unfortunately, they did not indicate whether the subjects themselves believed this or whether this belief related to others: a crucial point.

Some authors make passing reference to staff using seclusion as a means of punishment but tend not to dwell on the topic, and provide little evidence other than personal views. For example, ' . . . the fact that punitive motives on the part of the staff may occasionally precipitate seclusion of such patients cannot be totally overlooked' (Ramchandani, Akhtar and Helfrich, 1981);

'the unit's list of reasons for seclusion offers some evidence that seclusion at times is used as a weapon of retaliation and control' (Binder, 1979); and the use of seclusion because of ' ... staff resentment at non-compliance' (Soloff, 1987). There is also some suggestion that the duration of seclusion is closely related to the affronting of staff dignity at the time of the crisis (Binder, 1979).

As we stated earlier, relatively scant reference is made in the literature to the notion of punishment as a motivation for seclusion, possibly due to the depth of feeling engendered by staff who feel themselves professionally above and beyond any such actions. However, if we are to move forwards in our understanding of the seclusion issue we must broach this subject in an objective and intelligent manner, and if we cannot, then it most certainly does not augur well for the future of psychiatric care.

If we are analysing human behaviour in terms of rape, murder and arson, which in forensic psychiatry we do daily, then we should at least be able to attempt to analyse and examine the revenge factor in relation to seclusion use. Without this examination we will be left with the platitudinal facade of staff verbalizing seclusion use as therapeutic, and will ' ... couch disciplinary measures in terms of patients' own best interests' (Gentilin, 1987).

Gair (1984) discussed the possibility of sadistic tendencies in nursing staff as a motivation for the use of seclusion, and argued that there was a need for constant review and investigation regarding prolonged seclusion use. We could find no research studies in our literature review that report such sadistic tendencies. Notwithstanding this, we are left with the catalogue of public inquiries down the years and the allegations therein, some upheld, some not, to augment this possibility. However, some nursing staff have admitted to acts of abuse which can only be described as cruel and sadistic. Perhaps this should not surprise us: when all is said and done, nursing staff are human, with all the human failings, and not, as the public would have us believe, divine guardians.

5

Legal aspects and policy issues

Tom Mason

Issues tend to become contentious due to personal, professional, political and legal considerations, or a combination of all four, which would rightly suggest a complex structure to the issue under investigation. Nowhere is this more the case than with the topic of seclusion.

Up to the beginning of the 1980s there were very few journal articles regarding the seclusion of the psychiatric patient, but during that decade the number of articles increased significantly, with the trend appearing to continue into the 1990s (Figure 5.1). There could be many reasons for this increased interest. It may be that professional practitioners began an increased examination of seclusion spontaneously, at the turn of the 1980s, out of academic interest; or it may have been due to a heightened moral appreciation of the concern to improve patient care that provided the spark. It could possibly have been the result of the western shift towards consumerism or the drifting imagery of postmodern thought. However, it would appear to us that one of the main reasons why the seclusion issue lay dormant for so long was more likely to have been related to the lack of public awareness. However, this changed towards the end of the 1970s and in the early 1980s, with clinicians and hospital administrators finding themselves embroiled in litigation, with lawsuits brought by patients who had been secluded and restrained.

It is questionable whether without such litigation seclusion would have come under such close scrutiny as it did, but we would not totally agree with Soloff (1987), who argued that 'Were

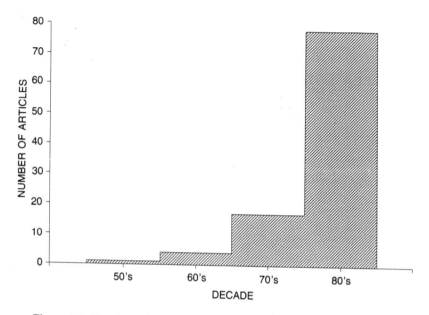

Figure 5.1 Number of published articles relating to seclusion

it not for psychiatry's legal critics, seclusion and restraint in the modern treatment milieu most certainly would have remained unstudied'.

THE BOSTON STATE CASE

On 29 October 1979, Federal District Court Judge Joseph Tauro adjudged that patients in Massachusetts had the right to refuse treatment, which included seclusion, in the case of non-emergency situations. This was in response to seven patients filing suit to stop the use of medication (non-emergency) of voluntary and involuntary patients at the Boston State Hospital in 1975. The decision itself caused a 'continuing clinicolegal conundrum' (Mills, 1981) which remains extant today.

The legal debate centred around whether seclusion was in response to violent outbursts and used as a means of containment, or whether it represented a method of treating an underlying illness. It would appear that these diametrically opposed positions constitute the medicolegal non-alignment so often seen in the literature on seclusion. The fundamental legal question at issue was whether a patient had the right to refuse medication in non-emergency situations. The plaintiffs' argument was that seclusion was not a form of treatment but a punishment which was used wilfully, for arbitrary durations, and without due consideration for the rights of patients. The defence claimed that seclusion was a respected form of treatment which many disturbed patients found valuable and was necessary for the safety of all during psychiatric emergencies.

Applebaum and Gutheil (1980) suggested that the misuse and misunderstanding of the concept of psychotropic medication, often used as an adjunct to seclusion, along with the prosecution's use of emotive terms such as 'involuntary mind control' to describe its effects, were central to the court's conclusions, and that 'moreover, the language reveals no sense that it is truly the illness and not the treatment that deserves the label' (Applebaum and Gutheil, 1980). The forced use of medication while a patient was in seclusion was deemed unacceptable by the court on the grounds that since the patient was already being restrained by seclusion the refusal to take medication would not have precipitated an emergency. They argued: 'The clear implication is that if a patient is being given one form of emergency treatment (seclusion) he cannot be given another form of emergency treatment (involuntary medication) at the same time . . . ' (Gutheil, 1980). A major problem here is whether seclusion is seen only as a restraint technique or as a treatment modality. It would appear that Judge Tauro believed the former to be the case, as can be seen in his adjudication, whereas Mills (1981) argued for the latter.

The problem of psychotropic medication usage overlapped considerably with seclusion in the court's deliberations, and it appears that they attached to the function of this medication the prime rationale of 'mind altering', not in the sense of controlling the psychiatric symptoms but as a contravention of the First Amendment as regards the patient's right to produce and communicate his own thoughts. The court's separation of seclusion and medication as independent responses to emergencies showed little appreciation of multiple approaches sometimes used with extremely disturbed individuals. Mills (1981) highlighted this point: 'For adequate behavioural control, some patients require all three restraints, physical, chemical and seclusion'. By raising this question of the level of restrictiveness it implies that seclusion is not a therapeutic intervention but merely a form of control. If this be so, then it is a matter of personal interpretation as to what form of control is most restrictive. If a person's behaviour requires controlling, what method would be least constraining: chemicals, physical restraints or a seclusion room? It is, of course, recognized that some establishments may use a combination of restraints and, in a few cases, all three at the same time.

However, if it is argued that seclusion is a treatment modality then the hierarchical restrictiveness debate is somewhat laid to rest, as it now becomes an issue of the individual clinical needs of the patient. Quite clearly, if a patient responds better to one drug rather than another, given the side effects, then he would be prescribed the former rather than an alternative. Similarly, it can be argued that if a person responds better to seclusion, rather than medication, the former would be given (given the facilities) rather than the latter. This, it is emphasized, is the case only if it is accepted that seclusion is viewed as a therapeutic intervention. Many do not accept this rationale.

Whatever else the Boston State case may have been responsible for, it is fair to suggest that 'The concern of psychiatry's critics and the resulting judicial reviews have prompted renewed interest in systematic studies on the use of seclusion and restraint in the modern treatment milieu, (Soloff, 1987). This is evidenced by the number of articles published on the topic of seclusion since the case in question.

OTHER CASES

The Boston State case was not the only litigation that had an influence on the scrutiny of seclusion use. The case of *Youngberg V Romeo*, also in America, in 1982, was centred around the case of a severely mentally impaired man, Romeo, who was committed to a State School Hospital in Pennsylvania. Romeo, according to Wexler (1982), was an extremely violent man, both to himself and to other residents, who would react against him and cause him injuries. Romeo claimed an infringement to his constitutional rights and sued for damages on the grounds that he had a ' ... constitutional right to safety, to freedom of movement and to training' (Wexler, 1982).

Although the Supreme Court ruled that patients were constitutionally entitled to personal safety and freedom from physical restraints, these rights were extensively curtailed by the court. As for the right to training, the court felt it necessary to interpret Romeo's right more painstakingly. The court recognized the conflict inherent in the right to bodily safety of a patient who is being attacked by another patient, and also the right of bodily freedom for the attacker. The answer to this obvious dilemma was to equivocate on these rights and make the decision on what was termed professional judgement. However, despite the protracted adjudication the solution to these complex issues remained unresolved.

In Britain, seclusion has featured large in many inquiry reports from both the general psychiatric facilities and the special hospitals.

During the 1980s there have been three deaths of patients while in seclusion at Broadmoor. In the first, in July 1984, the patient died through aspirating his vomit. The postmortem concluded that the pre-disposing factors to the patient's death were (a) excitement and high emotions associated with psychiatric disturbance and violent struggles; (b) a period of cerebral hypoxia caused by the compression to the neck (allegedly caused during the initial incident which resulted in the seclusion); (c) recent ingestion of a considerable quantity of confectionery prior to the disturbance; and (d) the use of sodium amytal and sparine, alone or in combination (Ritchie, 1985).

The second death in seclusion, in August 1988, occurred when an extremely violent man was deemed to require sedation while in the seclusion room armed with a weapon fashioned from a pair of broken glasses lost by a member of staff during the original struggle. A control and restraint team was organized and, using protective helmets and shields, the nursing staff were able to restrain the violent patient and administer 200 mg of chlorpromazine. It is reported that within 2 minutes of the seclusion room being vacated the patient was observed to be motionless. A verdict of accidental death was returned (Atha, 1989).

The third case is still under investigation and the final report is, as yet, unavailable.

Broadmoor is not the only special hospital where patients have died while in seclusion. Ashworth Special Hospital (formerly Moss Side and Park Lane) was subject to a public inquiry in 1991/92 which included an investigation into the death of a patient while in seclusion in March 1988. The patient was taken to the seclusion room following an altercation with a member of staff at 8.10 p.m. and was kept there overnight. In the morning the seclusion continued until approximately 12.30 p.m. when the patient collapsed and was pronounced dead some 20 minutes later. The postmortem reported that the cause of death was unascertainable from the autopsy. In the inquiry report the role of the drug pimozide was brought into question. Unfortunately, however, the dangerous side effects of this drug were not known until 1990.

Seclusion featured large in the Ashworth Inquiry Report, which investigated allegations of physical, sexual and chemical abuse of patients while in seclusion (Blom-Cooper, 1992).

Rampton Special Hospital has also recently (May 1992) had a patient die in seclusion, the Judge deciding that accidental death was the appropriate finding.

Of course, the deaths of patients while in seclusion do not only occur in the special hospitals; indeed, Nelson *et al.* (1983) reported the '..unusual death of a patient in seclusion' in a mental hospital in Pennsylvania. The patient, diagnosed as suffering from paranoid schizophrenia, had become assaultative and extremely bizarre in his thoughts and behaviour. At the time the patient was prescribed thiothixene, a major tranquillizer with side effects similar to those of chlorpromazine, 20 mg twice daily. The second dose of thiothixene was given at 4 p.m. and at 6.45 p.m. the patient was observed to be lying under his vinyl-covered mattress which, the authors state, was unvented and made of foam. At 7 p.m., having torn the outer cover of the mattress, the patient was noted to be lying, head first, between the outer vinyl and the inner foam, motionless. He was pronounced dead at 7.07 p.m.

Deaths in mental hospitals, let alone in seclusion, have a historical image of bizarre mystification, notwithstanding the scientific explanations given in accounts. In a report from Massachusetts, in 1980, there were 40 unexpected deaths over a 3-year period in the public mental facilities in that state, of which more than 20 were unexplained. The cases included a patient who was evidently tied to a tree and burned to death, and another case involved a female patient who disappeared without a trace except for seven teeth found in the possession of another patient (Des Moines Register, 1980). The report confirmed that not only were the deaths unexplained, but that they were not investigated thoroughly by either the Mental Health Department or other appropriate agencies. This is not specific to these cases from Massachusetts, as reports from around the world highlight a similar state of affairs. However, the statement from Senator Jack Backman regarding the report could speak for many institutions and mental health services: 'widespread violations of state laws and regulations as well as major deficiencies in treatment planning and patient care are common in Massachusetts programs for the mentally ill . . . in particular, we found that seclusion, chemical and mechanical restraints were frequently used without justification' (Des Moines Register, 1980).

MENTAL HEALTH ACT, CODE OF PRACTICE AND SECLUSION

The Mental Health Act (MHA) of England and Wales (HMSO, 1983) is extremely ambiguous and subject to extensive variability of interpretation in relation to the use of seclusion. The Code of Practice pertaining to the MHA 1983 is not. Confusingly, the two documents appear at odds with each other over the issue of seclusion.

The Code of Practice informs us (page 77) that seclusion falls within the definition of 'medical treatment' under Section 145 of the MHA 1983. In true judicial parlance, Section 145 interprets 'medical treatment' as being inclusive of 'nursing . . . care, habilitation and rehabilitation under medical supervision' (HMSO, 1983). However, the 'treatment' of a patient is covered by Section 3 of the MHA 1983. In this section there is a particular focus on three aspects of treatment. First, that the patient is suffering from a form of mental disorder categorized by the MHA; secondly, that treatment is likely to alleviate or prevent a deterioration in the condition; and thirdly, that it is necessary for the health and safety of the patient or for the protection of others that he should receive such treatment (Gostin, 1983). The treatability requirement was a fundamental shift away from mere custodianship, focusing on the specifics of alleviation of a condition or, at the very least, the prevention of a deterioration. If seclusion is to fall within this legal framework as a 'medical treatment', which as we have already seen is extremely dubious, it must satisfy the criteria of being either a therapy or a means of containment (see Chapter 4).

However, the Code of Practice is unambiguous: ' . . . seclusion is not a treatment technique and should not feature as part of any treatment programme' (HMSO, 1990). This eliminates any therapeutic rationale for the use of seclusion and makes it perfectly clear that it is **not** a treatment modality. The Code of Practice goes on to state that the use of seclusion cannot be anticipated and should not be used because of reduced staffing levels. This clearly advocates the use of seclusion as an emergency measure in response to a clinical crisis. Seclusion use, therefore, cannot feature as part of a care plan, although obviously when seclusion is implemented as an emergency a care plan is called for. The Code of Practice argues that seclusion is totally inappropriate for use with suicidal patients, or where there is a threat of self-injurious behaviours. They conclude that ' . . . its sole aim therefore is to contain severely disturbed behaviour which is likely to cause harm to others' (HMSO, 1990). As the code also unequivocally affirms that seclusion should not be used as a form of punishment, or as a mechanism to enforce appropriate behaviours, it can be seen that the only rationale for seclusion falls within the containment principle.

The discrepancy between the MHA's and the Code of Practice's patently clear positions regarding seclusion can be interpreted on two distinct levels. First, it can be suggested that the 7 years between the documents, and their divergent positions, could be regarded as constitutive of a fundamental shift in the theoretical rationale for seclusion which, if true, is a remarkable change of opinion in such a relatively short period of time. Secondly, the conflicting opinions could be indicative of the function that each document serves to maintain. The MHA is a statutory piece of legislation and, as such, it becomes the law of the land by which courts must rule on any given practice, whereas the Code of Practice offers guiding principles and articles of faith based on ideals of what the best practice would constitute. This allows for a much freer interpretation, although it must also be stressed that although the Code of Practice does not delegate a legal responsibility it can be referred to in legal proceedings.

A major concern in the MHA's suggestion that seclusion is a form of medical treatment is that the detained patient then has a right to withdraw consent. Although it is appreciated that seclusion does not fall within 'surgical operations' or 'administration of medicine', it clearly does constitute 'medical treatment for mental disorder' by its own definition (HMSO, 1983). This is despite Section 63 of the MHA, stating that the consent of a patient is not required for medical treatment if given by, or under the direction of, the responsible medical officer. In reality, although the responsible medical officer may sanction the use of seclusion they invariably have little else to do with it.

Despite the fact that seclusion use is not directly related to the nurse's holding power (MHA 1983, Section 5 (4)) a brief mention will be made. The MHA states that a psychiatric inpatient can be detained against their will for a maximum of 6 hours if the patient ' . . . is suffering from a mental disorder to such a degree that it is necessary for his health or safety or for the protection of others for him to be immediately restrained from leaving the hospital . . . ' (HMSO, 1983). Under statute it is questionable whether secluding a patient fitting the above criteria is justifiable, although physically restraining the patient appears legitimate.

In British common law a nurse (or any other person) can apprehend and restrain a person who is mentally disordered if it is believed that they represent a danger to themselves or others. Although these powers are not embodied in statute, an individual is entitled to restrain another person in an emergency and, as Gostin (1983) has pointed out, 'this could mean physically controlling the patient by bodily force or mechanical restraints or seclusion'. It is emphasized, of course, that these common law powers are extremely limited: they can only be used in the case of an immediate danger and the degree and duration must be very carefully measured.

We can see, throughout this study on seclusion, that the legal aspects and the policy issues vacillate between ideology, legislation and pragmatics. This is understandable, given that mental disorder, dangerousness and the need to protect are as old as mankind itself.

ROYAL COLLEGE OF NURSING, ROYAL COLLEGE OF PSYCHIATRISTS AND SECLUSION

In a paper entitled 'Seclusion and Restraint in Hospitals and Units for the Mentally Disordered' (RCN, 1979) the Royal College of Nursing were very concerned about the apparent lack of guidelines for the use of seclusion and restraint, and perturbed that Regional Health Authorities lacked comprehensive policies specific to their use. They were also alarmed that at a clinical level there were considerable discrepancies between what was occurring in practice and what the scantily worded policies had written down.

The Royal College of Nursing went to some considerable length in attempting to correct this very obvious policy and procedural gap by producing a general overview of what should constitute a *modus operandi*. They highlighted the procedural issues, which included attention to the safety of the patient during seclusion and restraint and the necessity of appropriate observation and assessment of behaviour. They also focused on the role of research in these issues, taking into account the need for appropriate ward design and relevant facilities to be made available. The RCN document also pointed out that the seclusion review procedure should incorporate a 2- and 4-hourly review policy. The detailed recording of the seclusion was listed and the importance of the patients rights was also emphasized. The rights of staff were covered and protection advised under the Mental Health Act 1959 (HMSO, 1959), the Criminal Law Act 1967 (HMSO, 1967) and under common law defence. They concluded with comments regarding chemical, physical and mechanical restraint (RCN, 1979). Considering that this document predates the Mental Health Act 1983 by 4 years and the Code of Practice 1990 by 11, it stood as a leading text on seclusion and restraint ahead of its time. The later Code of Practice contains many of the policy suggestions discussed in it.

The Royal College of Nursing reviewed and updated their guidelines in 1992 and, prior to outlining the procedure for seclusion use, they discussed the contemporary issues relating to seclusion. These included the types of behaviours that can contribute to management problems and the possible causes of problem behaviours. General preventative measures were highlighted, with a particular emphasis on adequate staffing levels as well as the development of skill and expertise of nursing staff. The 1992 document was also concerned over the increased number of violent incidents that have been reported and the development of control and restraint techniques. However, a cautionary note was heard when they emphasized that these 'techniques should not be viewed in isolation from existing therapeutic, interventional skills' (RCN, 1992). The role of education in the management of violent incidents featured large, and possible areas for curriculum development were pointed out.

The importance of these two documents was not so much that they took on board the contemporary issues relating to seclusion, which in fact is very important, it was that they were written at a very practical level with a focus on the real issues dealing with violent incidents. They were, and are, documents for the practitioners.

In contrast, the Royal College of Psychiatrists (RCP) have paid very scant reference to the use of seclusion and restraint, and what is worse is that the early attention was both poor in quality and paternalistically condescending. For example, 'it is known that some psychiatric nurses have real conscience problems with regard to the need and justification for the provision of isolation facilities in psychiatric units; these feelings need to be taken into consideration' (RCP, 1981). This document was produced in response to a request from the General Nursing Council for England and Wales for the Royal College of Psychiatrists to consider whether psychiatric wards that practised seclusion were suitable for nurse training. We do not wish to dwell on whether such a request was appropriate, but rather to focus on the impoverished nature of the text. The RCP (1981) are at pains to blame nurses' questioning of the use of seclusion and restraint on their 'inexperience', 'lack of insight', 'narrow perception' and reduced level of 'knowledge if not skill'. This type of medical arrogance is misplaced in modern academic circles.

In the following year the Royal College of Psychiatrists (1982) produced another bulletin, 'Locking up patients by themselves', but this too was of a very limited quality. Preoccupied, once again, with demonstrating medical superiority, the document attempts to provide a framework of 'support and guidance of nurses', but fails to be convincing (RCP, 1982). The document goes on to present the procedure for the seclusion of patients in the Bethlem Royal and Maudsley Hospitals, which one can only assume is presented as the RCP's exemplar of a seclusion procedure. Unfortunately, by 1982 this was hopelessly out of date, and the constructs of the procedure appear primitive even by the RCN's standards some 3 years earlier.

The RCP's (1990) document was much better. In this, the College began addressing at least some of the issues pertaining to seclusion, such as staff deployment, design of seclusion rooms and the review procedure, and although it is not a comprehensive document it does perhaps reflect the importance of seclusion to the medical profession. It is interesting to note that the majority of writers on seclusion in Britain are nurses, which possibly demonstrates that, as nurses bear the brunt of operating a seclusion procedure, it is of greater import as a nursing issue.

HEALTH AUTHORITIES AND SECLUSION

Leopoldt (1985) reported that from a survey of 42 psychiatric hospitals, seven had definite non-seclusion policies and the remaining 35 used seclusion, albeit infrequently. From these 35 Leopoldt and his co-workers had access to 28 written seclusion policies. Although he reported that a relatively large number of hospitals had recently reviewed and updated their policies and procedures, he also noted a wide variance of content between the documents.

Prior to the 1959 Mental Health Act and the sweeping re-organization of the NHS in the 1960s, the regulation and recording of seclusion in psychiatric hospitals was undertaken uniformly, and was the sole responsibility of the medical superintendent. However, following the reorganization it was left to each individual hospital and/or health authority to decide whether seclusion should be used, whether policies were required and what mechanism of recording should be undertaken, if any. This has now led to a situation in which there is no uniformity of practice, policy, recording or communication regarding seclusion. There is no network of policies between Health Authorities and very little flow of information between hospitals. This has driven the issue underground to an ominous and secretive level, which has proved most unhelpful in attempting to examine the subject.

The question arises as to what constitutes the operational practices of seclusion if no official guidelines exist, and how these practices are learned. Much knowledge regarding seclusion is communicated at an informal level, based on past experiences which are disseminated via anecdotes and stories that form part of the institutional mythology. Part of the trouble with this approach is that stories become embellished and enriched with the passage of time, and the issue takes on new dimensions and features, which makes scientific research and exploration into the subject fraught with sensitivities. It is perhaps not surprising, therefore, that seclusion use is sometimes surrounded with silence.

This lack of official channels for reviewing the use of seclusion has produced an inconsistent and haphazard approach, which appears to stumble from scandal to scandal and from inquiry to inquiry. However, it may also be argued that the production of guidelines, policies and procedures relating to seclusion not only sanctions its use but also establishes a certain legitimacy. The problem is, of course, a question of balance. Is it better to have no policy and hope that illicit seclusions do not occur? Or is it better to have open and frank guidelines and risk an increase in seclusion usage?

Another problem area in the policy issue is that because an 'official' policy exists it becomes almost sacred and thus unquestionable. It is a similar situation to a law that becomes statutory: once in place it is extremely difficult to change, and sometimes very difficult even to question its use. Even bad laws become accepted and appear to be almost incontestable. Seclusion policies should incorporate a powerful review mechanism and identify people responsible for examining its practice and a strategy for regulation.

In the main it falls to managers to formulate the policies, procedures and guidelines relating to seclusion, and great care is needed in grounding such policies in both practice requirements and conceptual frameworks. Managers, if not careful, can produce guidelines merely because nurses practice seclusion, with little real thought as to whether it is useful or even necessary. If the sole motivation for the production of guidelines is a legal imperative, then it is likely to have little room for progress, development and change.

HEALTH AND SAFETY AT WORK AND SECLUSION

The Health and Safety at Work Act (1974), Section 2(2)e states that it is the employer's duty to ensure 'the provision and maintenance of a working environment for his employees that is, so far as is reasonably practicable, safe, without risks to health, and adequate as regards facilities and arrangements for their welfare at work' (HMSO, 1974). Clearly, this could include safe working policies regarding the management of violent incidents, and may also incorporate the provision of seclusion facilities in the event of staff being at risk of injury. It is certainly the case that it is the duty of the employing authority to provide 'such information, instruction, training and supervision as is necessary to ensure, so far as is reasonably practicable, the health and safety at work of his employees' (HMSO, 1974). Therefore, it is clearly the responsibility of managers to educate and inform staff regarding the management of violent behaviours and not merely leave those at the clinical frontier to fend for themselves, with inadequate guidelines and poor support mechanisms. It is relatively easy to issue impractical policy statements from the safe comfort of an office desk while ignoring the stress, fears and anxieties of those who have to deal with the extremes of violent behaviours.

There is, of course, the stress factor to be taken into consideration in any non-seclusion policy. If there are no alternative strategies to prevent injuries to staff and other patients, then the employing authority is at fault in not safeguarding the welfare of those in their charge: welfare facilities are regarded as part of the overall working environment, and if reasonable steps are not taken to prevent staff being assaulted then employing authorities are liable. As Broadhurst (1978) pointed out, 'it is the practice, at least at common law, to regard some activities which might be deemed 'welfare matters' as reasonably incidental to a person's employment so that these would presumably be included within the term welfare'.

The Health and Safety at Work Act (1974), Section 1(3), unambiguously states that an employer should not put at risk any persons by asking them to undertake an action which is part of the nature of the organization's function, which is related to the materials used, or if the condition of the premises is unsatisfactory. The function of a psychiatric hospital is, of course, in part the management of disturbed behaviour, and the materials used are often human. Yet the Act clearly states that there is a duty to minimize risks to the organization's employees. This needs careful thought when a reduction or elimination of seclusion is considered.

QUALITY ASSURANCE AND SECLUSION

In much of the literature on seclusion, reference is made to the necessity of reducing its use, in both frequency and duration. This appears somewhat paradoxical, in that if it is therapeutic then a reduction in therapy appears to be contraindicated unless there is a comparative reduction in the 'disease', but the aim should always be to use the minimum therapeutic dose. The problem with the level of seclusion use and quality assurance initiatives is similar to the prescribing of medication in relation to budgetary considerations. Ideally, we would like to think that the right drug in the right quantities would be prescribed irrespective of cost. However, in the real world this is not always the case.

If seclusion has a high profile in a particular hospital and is linked to quality assurance indicators, the values underpinning its use will change. Measuring seclusion figures as a level of performance brings pressures to bear which may produce a reduced level of seclusion but may also produce hidden consequences. Illicit seclusionary practices may be adopted, staff and other patients may be put at risk, and an increase in medication and restraints is a possible corollary. It may be that the production of a graph indicating the decreasing use of seclusion is proudly presented and received with high regard, but a much more rigorous analysis and incisive enquiry is required if the project is not to sink into the abyss of another 'platitudinal facade' (Mason and Chandley, 1990).

The factors surrounding seclusion use continue to be measured as an indicator of both scientific inquiry and as a description of meaning. Unfortunately, this misses the basic point, which is the experience of the patients who undergo seclusion, their perceptions of the isolation and what it means to them, both during the episode and its long-term effects. This has to be contrasted with the feelings of staff who have to deal with the possibility of assault without the skills, resources or mechanisms for extricating themselves from potentially dangerous situations.

PATIENTS' CHARTER AND SECLUSION

Within the framework of the government's Patients' Charter, including the Citizens' Charter, and both the National Charter Standards and Local Charter Standards, there are a number of issues concerning seclusion.

First, there is patient advocacy, which involves each patient having a direct link with an independent person who can support him and speak on his behalf in his best interests. In relation to seclusion, the patient's advocate could become part of the assessment process and there may be a role for them in the review procedures. They could also act on behalf of the patient in seclusion debriefing sessions, if the patient was incapable, whether or not they agreed with his views, otherwise the fundamental relationship between the patient and the advocate would be put in jeopardy. (Advocacy is discussed in Chapter 8.)

A second issue is the role of the named nurse, who will have a special interest in and knowledge of the patient. Such systems as primary and secondary nursing and key workers have been in vogue for many years now, but the named nurse approach means that every patient should have this facility. There is a very obvious role for the named nurse in the use of seclusion, as knowledge of the patient, particularly in times of crisis, is vital for assessment purposes.

The third issue to emerge is the complaints procedure. As from 1 April 1992 it became a right 'to have any complaint about NHS services, whoever provides them, investigated, and to receive a full and prompt written reply from the chief executive of your health authority or general manager of your hospital' (HMSO, 1992). The complaints procedure is a vital mechanism for ensuring that the rights of patients are protected. This is always important, but takes on crucial proportions when it concerns compulsory confinement of a patient behind a locked door. It is as much about protecting the staff as it is about safeguarding the patient. Patients should always have avenues of complaint which can be used positively to air grievances, review standards and assess care delivery.

EUROPEAN CONVENTION ON HUMAN RIGHTS AND SECLUSION

Article 3 provides that 'No one shall be subjected to torture or to inhumane or degrading treatment or punishment' (Jacobs, 1975), and there are no exceptions or restrictions. Since its drafting in 1948, there have been thousands of allegations examined under this article, and although many refer to such atrocities as electric shocks, mock executions and threats to kill, some have dealt with seclusion, physical restraints and solitary confinement.

In Zeidler–Kornman vs Federal Republic of Germany, prison officers who had severely handled a prisoner and placed him in a straitjacket were charged with inhuman and degrading treatment under Article 3. The Commission found no evidence of injury and concluded that this did not amount to inhuman and degrading treatment. It also noted that the reason for the use of the straitjacket was the prisoner's violent behaviour.

Although the Commission have found that the use of solitary confinement is undesirable, they have been loth to suggest that it violates Article 3. 'Thus the Commission has rejected as being manifestly ill-founded, on the particular facts, complaints of detention in solitary confinement' (Jacobs, 1975). They have, however, been concerned with the conditions of the confinement and its length in individual cases.

However, the European Commission of Human Rights did adopt a report in July 1980, in which the complainant had alleged that he had been treated in a degrading and inhumane manner while receiving treatment as a patient in Broadmoor Special Hospital. This alleged abuse involved being secluded for 5 weeks in 1974 because, he claimed, he was suspected of setting a fire on one of the wards. The case was never adjudicated upon, as the patient concerned accepted a friendly settlement which included, among other things, a requirement for new guidelines on seclusion to be instigated at Broadmoor. Other than a general review within the, then, four special hospitals for England and Wales, this case had little impact on changing seclusion practice.

In conclusion, the legal ramifications of seclusion practice are far-reaching and complex. This means that the decision to use seclusion is an extremely important one to make, not only for the patient but also for the staff responsible for that decision.

6

Decision-making process in seclusion practice

Tom Mason

Much of nursing practice, and indeed everyday life, is based on making choices from sets of alternatives that are presented to us. These choices can be made actively or passively. For example, we make choices regarding how we are going to get out of bed in the morning, what clothes we are going to wear and how we are going to dress ourselves. Some people select the time they are going to get out of bed on a daily basis, weighing up how they feel each morning and what they want to do once they are up. Others make a predetermined choice, in that they automatically arise the moment the alarm sounds. In other words it has become their routine to do this.

Another example is the choice of clothes that one is going to wear each morning. Some make an active choice from a number of garments in the wardrobe, whereas others have a uniform set of working clothes. Although when we were learning to dress ourselves as toddlers we may have actively chosen which foot we were going to place our shoe on first, in adulthood this is no longer a consideration: it has become routinized.

So it is with nursing practice and, more specifically, with the decision whether or not to use seclusion.

CULTURAL AND ORGANIZATIONAL CONSTRUCTS

It must be said from the outset that the development of habits is essential to free our information-processing capacities. Otherwise we would probably not have time for the more important activities of life (Bourne *et al.*, 1986). However, part of the problem of decision-making is that if we are choosing from the same set of alternatives each time, and the same choice has been successful for us before, then we are likely to continue with that choice each time and eventually it becomes habitual. If this choice involves others and what happens to them, then it is important to assess the complete set of alternatives on each occasion.

The decision-making process takes place within the cultural and organizational frameworks in which we are operating at the time. This means that we may make decisions that we might not make in another sphere of life. The organization and its culture, therefore, determines how we arrive at decisions regarding practice. Psychiatric institutions have their own culture, philosophy and value systems and to understand more fully the decision-making process in any of these settings we need to analyse their roles and culture. As we are focusing on the decision whether or not to use seclusion, we turn our attention to the cultural framework in which that decision takes place.

Control

The controlling nature of our society has been well documented by writers such as Foucault (1980) and Cohen (1985), and indeed, without control we would soon deteriorate into chaos. However, control can take on ominous characteristics when it becomes institutionalized and the power to control is invested in the vagaries of human nature. It would be nice to think that rules governing practice, mental health acts, hospital policies and codes of conduct are such that those operating degrees of control do not go beyond the boundaries of decree, but in all walks of life there are those who breach the rules. An interesting point here is that many of those who would contravene a practice regulation, for example secluding a patient for retributive reasons, believe that they are right and just in that decision, their rationale being that it is in the patient's best interests in the long run (Mason, 1992).

Psychiatry itself has come under close scrutiny as a measure of social control (Szasz, 1974). Szasz illuminates the notion that psychiatry and the law are enmeshed in a fundamental social need to control human beings who are considered aberrant. Certainly parallels can be drawn between the investigative approaches of the police, the examination of evidence in the courts, the psychiatric interview and psychoanalysis, and the idea that certain nursing practices, within the field of forensic psychiatry, amount to a form of 'societal policing' was reported by Mason and Chandley (1990). The thrust of the argument was that the identification of psychiatric symptoms in forensic inpatients serves to reinforce the perpetuation of their compulsory detention.

If the role of the psychiatric nurse incorporates such constructs as the learnt behaviours from such value systems as control, surveillance, investigation and policing, then it is not too difficult to understand why psychiatric institutions breed hierarchies of dominance. Goffman's excellent work in this area is testimony to the subtle ways in which hospitals develop hierarchies of dominance and a whole societal system of control, power, surveillance and punishment. The use of the privilege system can lead to all manners of abuse; Goffman's argument is that 'the very notions of punishments and privileges are not ones that are cut from civilian cloth' (Goffman, 1968). Goffman goes to some length in setting out the depersonalizing nature of the total institution, the career of the mental patients within that institution, and the strategies they employ to survive the formal and informal rules of the institution. He makes no suggestions as to how alternatives to the power, control and dominance aspects of total institutions may be organized, but provides an excellent portrayal of the institutional social mechanisms that were extant at that time and the function they served in maintaining the social order of the institution.

Unfortunately, Goffman does not inform us as to how large groups of people should be controlled, if indeed they should, and no reference is made to the controlling mechanisms of the wider society, such as the law and the police.

In a study of psychiatric settings in America, Eileen Morrison (1990) identified the 'tradition of toughness' as a key concept that dominated the culture. From the 'cultural family' constructs that she identified, a brief mention will be made of the following two categories. 'The need for physical restraint' category identified how new staff were socialized into accepting that the natural response to verbal outbursts was instant restraint, rather than giving time for other therapeutic activity. In this process any attempts by newcomers to delay the restraint by applying other alternatives were met with hostile comments from staff and the withdrawal of support on future occasions. This isolated the newcomer and suppressed any further attempts to change nursing practice in relation to the management of disturbed behaviour.

The second category, that of 'role component', identified three strategies that nursing staff employed in enforcing control over patients. First, 'policing', where staff saw themselves as experts in crisis intervention. Morrison offers one subject's description of this as 'the culture of toughness is based on the ideal of machismo; then, what you have is an increase in confrontation. When the value is placed on being tough, then you *handle* them' (Morrison, E., 1990). Secondly, 'supermanning' was identified as a strategy for those nursing staff who were physically the toughest of the enforcers. They were the ones who sanctioned physical aggression for controlling patients, which they did, quite effectively, when they were there. However, in her study Morrison described the problem being that 'when the 'superman' is not there everyone else's anxiety goes up' (Morrison, E., 1990). Thirdly, the strategy of 'putting on a show' was described as '...how the enforcers protect themselves from outside influences and negative sanctions for behaviour not officially condoned by the system' (Morrison, E., 1990). In this strategy nursing staff were adept at covering up their ulterior motives for their actions by providing 'textbook' rationales of nursing care delivery, which resulted in a professional facade.

This excellent study shows that the very human practice of nursing often does not corroborate the general perception that it is always ideally practised. From three psychiatric units under study, the cultural framework in which nurses were making decisions regarding the restraining of patients appeared to make it acceptable to base those decisions on the 'tradition of toughness'.

Although Morrison's study focused on restraints, the same argument may hold some truth for seclusion, and it is easy to see how the decision to use seclusion may have its roots deep within the culture of 'toughness'. When the object of a society is the control of humans, their behaviours and their thought processes, via psychiatry, it is perhaps not surprising that some of the controllers become aberrant.

Transgression of certain codes

The decision to seclude psychiatric patients is a very complex issue, and the decision not to seclude is equally complex. The reasons offered for the initiation of a seclusion regime often do not reflect the reasoning process that lies behind the decision. For example, it is easy to criticize such rationales for seclusion as 'refused medication', 'hostile', 'sarcastic', 'rude to staff', 'speech has violent content', and 'threw water or urine at staff' (Binder, 1979), and it is difficult to see any other reason than as retribution for the affront to staff feelings.

However, it may not be quite as clear-cut as that. If the patient's history is well known, or past behaviours have indicated that, for example, the violent content of a patient's conversation is a prodromal sign of an impending assault on another person, and alternative interventions have failed, then the reason offered takes a different aspect. What is particularly interesting is that, no matter what the reasons are, the person making the decision has undergone some process of thought and has judged that seclusion is the appropriate response. In short, they believe they are right in that decision. Whatever boundary the patient has crossed, whatever limit has been broken, the conclusion is that seclusion is right and proper. The fact that this goes against others' personal and professional codes is a matter of value judgement, despite the fact that sanctions may be brought against that particular staff member for transgressing someone else's code, for example the hospital's. This only serves to highlight that one value system has power (based on consensus) over another. It does not mean that the value system is in itself right and proper.

These value judgements, which affect the decision-making process, are developed through links with the wider society as well as professional ideologies, and serve to rationalize any number of nursing actions. As Ramchandani, Akhtar and Helfrich (1981) observe, ' . . . the fact that punitive motives on the part of the staff may occasionally precipitate seclusion of such patients cannot be totally overlooked'. Although it cannot be condoned, retribution is a well understood human motive, and when a person believes they have right on their side it can soon lead to conflicting sets of behaviours, which by their very nature are confrontational. It is this belief in the rightness of their actions which is their justification, and this brings us to the social communication of this rightness.

Media

The media also play their part in defining the value systems by which decisions are made regarding psychiatric practices. Television and newspapers form a large part of the communicative action that transmits certain values throughout society, evoking emotional responses from its members and monitoring their reactions. To paraphrase Jean Baudrillard: you do not only watch the television, the television also watches you, and you do not only read the newspapers, the newspapers also read you (Baudrillard, 1983). This two-way feedback mechanism was summed up by Kellner (1989): 'consequently on this view, the media pander to the masses, reproducing their taste, their interest in spectacle and entertainment, their fantasies and way of life . . . '. Seen in this light, the educational role of the media degenerates to the level of reinforcing events enacted by society.

Investigative journalism has become more and more acceptable in the postwar years, uncovering some of the great scandals of our time. The journalists become heroes as they battle against the massive bureaucracies of governments and large corporations, revealing cover-ups, corruption and malpractice. They are, in the main, applauded by society, and it is not until their intrusive trade probes individual lives that society begins to have doubts, although it must surely be of benefit when investigations unearth abuse and ill-treatment.

Some investigative journalism can be seen as little more than sensationalism, evoking readers' emotions, reaffirming and perpetuating them, in order to sell newspapers. This can be seen, for example, in headlines referring to forensic psychiatric patients, such as: 'Storm Over Bid to Free Sex Killer' (*Daily Mail*, 1985), and 'Monster in Shop Trip Horror' (*Sun*, 1989). The criticism is clear: these patients should not be allowed out of hospital; their offences warrant continued punishment by further incarceration, and it is acceptable for them to receive 'treatment' in a 'hospital' as long as the staff do not suggest that they are 'cured'. Contrast this with 'Mental Patients Terrified by Pig's Head at Repressive Hospital' (Brindle, 1992), in which the intention was to evoke pity for the vulnerable patients, who deserved kindness and compassion, and produce shock and disgust at nurses who break all the imagery of the devoted nurse administering relief from pain. A confusing media picture!

DECISION-MAKING THEORY

Decision-making has been studied from many perspectives; the following is a brief outline of some of the more favoured approaches to decision-making theory.

Expected-utility theory

This has been the dominant approach within decision-making theory for many years. However, recent refinements have produced differing versions which contain three central ideas:

1. The expected utility of an alternative is a weighted average of anticipated pleasures and pains.
2. Weights or probabilities and values are separate, but combine multiplicatively in determining expected utilities.
3. Choices are completely determined by expected utilities (Einhorn and Hogarth, 1981, cited by Bourne *et al.*, 1986).

Simply stated, this means that each alternative in any decision is evaluated in terms of its negative and positive aspects. When the expected utility of each alternative has been weighted, a choice is determined by the highest average (Table 6.1).

Table 6.1 Expected utilities averages for decision to seclude

	Seen to be in control	Safety of staff	Patient's interests	Revenge	Management preferences	Average expected utility
Seclusion	7	7	2	4	2	4.4
Non-seclusion	1	5	5	2	8	4.2
Alternative	3	5	4	3	6	4.2

Note: The factors in the decision are arbitrary ones as are the numbers which relate to a value for the decision maker. The higher number equates with a higher value.

In this scenario the decision would be made to seclude the patient, as the average expected utility for seclusion was highest. It must be stated that the factors relating to the decision would be individual to each decision-maker, and would consist of a range of features. However, this model assumes that each factor receives a value, and this averaging out determines the choice. This is not always the case in reality, as strength of belief in one decision factor can sometimes outweigh all the others.

Non-compensatory strategies

Whereas in the expected-utility approach the assessment of an alternative would involve an evaluation of all the factors' strengths and weaknesses, there are a number of decision strategies that are based on less than the full set of factors. Two will be briefly outlined.

According to the minimax strategy a comparison is made between the weakest values of decision factors, with the choice being the highest of the low scores. For example, in Table 6.1 an alternative to seclusion would be the chosen decision, as the lowest score of those factors is 3, whereas the lowest scores in the seclusion and non-seclusion choices are 2 and 1 respectively. The maximax strategy works in a similar manner but using the highest values among alternatives. The choice in this decision strategy would be non-seclusion, as the highest value is 8, with 7 and 6 for the other alternatives.

Decision conflict

Making an active choice takes time, and no matter how many alternatives are available prior to making the decision, once made, the selection options are usually much reduced. Whether the choice is made on the selection of positive factors or the rejection of negative ones matters only in relation to the expected outcome. In a number of decisions a time restriction may accompany the choice. However, some people attempt to reduce the dilemma of the decision by 'choosing not to choose' (Einhorn and Hogarth, 1981).

As Bourne *et al.* (1986) point out, any decision involves a cost, which can be negligible if one alternative dominates the others. However, in less clear decisions there may be a number of factors to be considered, and comparisons of alternatives which may be very close will result in a greater cost in deciding. The evidence would suggest that 'in a given situation, the benefit of choosing 'the best alternative' needs to be balanced against the cost of arriving at a decision' (Bourne *et al.*, 1986).

Heuristic strategies

It has been pointed out that people make decisions based on their own values; however, it must be added that these personal values will, in turn, be based on the norms of the social setting in which the decisions are made. Often decisions are made on the probability of things recurring, which will be based on past experiences. However, the laws of probability are much easier to assess than the reasoning of human beings. Take, for example, the representative heuristic strategy in which decisions may be made regarding the fiery temper of redheaded people or the social activity of blonde women. These types of fallacies can and do exist in our society, and provide the foundation for choices regarding these stereotypes. Suppose you meet four red-headed people who all lose their temper with you: what sort of decisions are you going to make about the fifth redheaded person you meet? And given the knowledge that there is no evidence to suggest that red-headed people are any more or less aggressive than other people, does that change your decision?

If you were asked to make a judgement regarding the number of words that begin with the letter r, and the number of words that have r in the third letter position, you would be more likely to judge that there are more words that begin with the letter r. This is because it is easier to recall such words than it is to remember words with r as the third letter. This is known as the availability heuristic. In fact, there are far more words with r as the third letter than as the first (Darley, Glucksberg and Kinchla, 1986).

These two heuristic strategies clearly show the weakness of human judgements in making everyday decisions, and it has been shown that when everyday practice becomes routine and commonplace, the conditions required for assessing and evaluating the flaws in human judgement are not established. This leads to a poor learning environment for developing better strategies, and most certainly does not provide a good grounding for producing change.

DECIDING ON SECLUSION: A RESEARCH EXAMPLE

An unpublished research study (Mason, 1989) was carried out in the late 1980s in a special hospital for England and Wales which caters for patients who require treatment under conditions of maximum security, due to their dangerous, violent or criminal propensities. Although a very appropriate environment to study the use of seclusion, the setting is a very difficult area in which to carry out this type of research. The main reason for this is the considerable overlap between psychiatry and criminology, which clouds the issue from both patient and staff points of view.

The nurses in this setting have conflicting views on their roles, which comprise on the one hand those aspects associated with care and compassion for the mentally afflicted, who require comfort, kindness and support within a professional relationship, and on the other hand the role of custodian, with the emphasis on security, containment and control, the ultimate violation of which is the escape of the patient.

The decision to initiate a seclusion regime in a special hospital falls to the nurse in charge at the time of the incident. At that point, the decision-maker affords him or herself an assessment which is complex, diverse and underpinned by an intricate reasoning process. The variation of decisions, in similar situations, highlights a diversity of individual choice which appears arbitrary and inconsistent. The fact that different nurses decide differently in similar situations makes it extremely difficult for patients to know what to expect.

Method and data collection

In a study of this nature the deep rooted personal feelings regarding the subject are overlaid with stringent legalized institutional policies and procedural guidelines. Coupled to this is the fact that the initiation of a seclusion regime following an incident is very much a response to an emergency situation which must be resolved quickly. This meant that certain traditional research techniques were unsuitable for the study.

The method employed was based on a phenomenological approach defined as the detailed description of conscious experience. This was undertaken by presenting each of the subjects with two typed scenarios of deteriorating ward situations, based upon which they were asked to make a decision regarding seclusion of the hypothetical patient. Once a decision had been made, the subjects were asked to give their rationale and considerations for it. Notes were taken and the subjects allowed to comment without prompting.

Interpretation of data

Following data collection from the 25 sample interviews, the content of each was analysed in terms of its practical reasoning; this analysis was then tape recorded and typed so that each discourse could be compared with the others.

The reasoning process appeared to be based in a historical–temporal framework, that is, the subjects analysed the immediate situation in terms of past experience, which is inextricably bound up with the notion of 'being' in the hospital as a social organization. Through their discourse the subjects showed their reasoning to be fixed within the hospital's socialization process, and responded to the problems presented in a consequential manner. This weighing up of the consequences of various lines of action was an integral part of their decision making.

The subject's 'life-world', to use Schutz's (1970) term, is based not only on his/her previous personal experience but also that of others which has been communicated to them. This is how the socialization process perpetuates a specific culture. The subject's reasoning is rooted in the totality of all past experiences, called 'the stock of knowledge' (Schutz, 1970), with the immediacy of the situation being dealt with from their own particular perception based on a historical analysis. Their own perception will reflect the values that have been communicated to them and which they have adopted as valuable.

There emerged three distinct operant themes that each subject underwent during the process of decision-making regarding seclusion. These were categorized as (a) mechanistic search, (b) frame conflict, (c) asylum status. In the mechanistic search mode the subjects presented alternative decisions in quick succession, with a rapid assessment of the consequences should the decision turn out to be the wrong one. They appeared to mentally present possible outcomes to the various scenarios and then rationalize away the alternatives, which would leave them with a confirmation of their own original decision on whether to seclude or not.

The second major theme to emerge, the frame conflict, emanated from the levels of stress caused by the dilemmas in the decision-making process or, more accurately, in the reasoning that underscores the decision. Through the mechanistic search the subjects became increasingly aware that they were in the 'frame', being seen by others or under someone's scrutiny, which appeared to create a conflict of operations. Although varying groups were identified as of some importance in the assessment of the subject's performance, all passed comment as to the existence of an 'audience' felt to be watching their decision.

The third theme to emerge was the positioning of the subject's decisions in a state of asylum, i.e. the adoption of a safety position. Subjects attempted to alleviate the future consequences of criticism by adopting a moral framework by which they could rebound their reasoning for their decision. The safest option was chosen.

At the point of deciding whether or not to seclude a patient, the subjects found that they perceived the immediate situation in terms of their unique personal history. This applied to all subjects in the study: their reasoning was fixed in the analysis of their 'stock of knowledge', which is constantly changing with the emergence of new experience. The constantly changing 'now' is referred to the stock of knowledge and grouped as 'familiar', 'same but modified' or 'strange'. This explains how a person deciding on seclusion perceives the present emerging situation, categorizes it and reflects back on previous successful strategies in dealing with that situation. This is likely to result in those previous successful strategies being applied to the current situation, and lead thence to the stagnation of practice relating to seclusion use.

A way forward is the adoption of two principles from the domain of action research, although both can be traced back to early Greek philosophy. The first principle is that of reflexivity. This is concerned with the ability of the human mind to reflect back on itself and engage in an analysis of its own subjective system of meanings. This is better developed in certain people than it is in others. Nonetheless, it is the potential for reflexivity which must be fostered. The reflexive process questions the usually accepted statements from oneself, opens up the verbal rationalizations of a discourse and can unearth deeper motives that organize and motivate our actions. One can never be totally sure what another person is thinking, and even our own thoughts are sometimes elusive. It is only by the process of questioning our own self that we can open up our minds to the possibilities that may be there. This leads to the second principle, that of dialectics.

Dialectics is concerned first with the conflict of meanings within argument, i.e. the dilemmas that exist in any dispute. Following on from the notion of reflexivity, it can be seen that the dialectical concern is with the conflict of interests that exist within ourselves; this can be related to the dilemma over whether to use seclusion or not. The dialectical concern would be with our own beliefs, prejudices, motives and rationalizations in relation to those of others. However, there is a second aspect of dialectics that needs to be mentioned, which is that it also encompasses the notion of progression, a way forwards through the dilemma: that by discussion, accepting the possibility of alternatives, opening up one's own thoughts to other points of view and analysing the conflict of interests, a new idea will emerge and an agreement can be made to put the new idea into practice. The new idea may not work, but what it will do is highlight new dilemmas, new conflicts and, hopefully, new ideas to try again.

Clearly, these principles stand in opposition to the stagnant, routinely operated decisions regarding the use of seclusion outlined at the beginning of the chapter, but it must be remembered that the principles of reflexivity and dialectics apply as much to those who argue against seclusion as to those who argue for its continuation.

In conclusion, the decision to use seclusion or not is theoretically complex, and rooted in the value systems of the professions, the institutions and their cultural framework. With the impetus being on the reduction of seclusion use and its ultimate eradication, there is a need to address the issues involved in non-seclusion policies.

7

Non-seclusion policies

Tom Mason and Ann Alty

There can be little doubt that initiatives in the field of mental health care are geared towards reducing the use of seclusion and eradicating it wherever possible. Even those who remain loyal to the belief that seclusion can be a therapeutic intervention advocate the reduction of its use, and that it should be used in extreme cases only. This is seen in much of the literature on seclusion, particularly those articles that reflect the personal views of those calling for its elimination. From those who attempt to defend its use there is always an air of anger and bitterness.

If we think carefully as to how and why seclusion was ever adopted as a method of dealing with psychiatric patients, and we accept the disentanglement that Chapter 4 hopefully achieved, then we are left with the core need to use seclusion, which is to prevent one human being from assaulting another. This appears to be the central aim of seclusion use.

When one is charged with the responsibility for managing patients who are disturbed and assaultative, this issue becomes of central importance. Where there is a non-seclusion policy, one must ask 'What has happened to the need to use seclusion?' and, 'How has the prevention of assault been achieved?'

Any non-seclusion policy must, first and foremost, deal with the issue of what is to be done with the patient who becomes assaultative when all else has failed. Remembering the old adage 'honesty is the best policy' is also a reasonable guiding principle when working towards eliminating seclusion. Far too often those who claim to use a non-seclusion policy merely hide its use from official view and submerge it in bad practice.

A survey carried out by Leopoldt (1985) while a member of

the Mental Health Act Commission produced information on 42 psychiatric hospitals, of which 35 used seclusion. It was claimed that 'seven had definite non-seclusion policies based on the principle that a seriously disturbed patient should not be left alone; although a single room for intensive nursing care was thought essential' (Leopoldt, 1985). What is not clear, however, is the nature of the 'seriously disturbed patient', and there is no mention as to how those hospitals managed the assaultative patient. One can only surmise that it was an unrealistic suggestion that nursing staff, left in the intensive care room with the disturbed patient, would allow themselves to be assaulted without resorting to curtailment in one form or another. Holding a patient down is clearly a form of restraint.

Leopoldt does pose the fundamental question that needs addressing in any non-seclusion policy, and hints at correlations between non-seclusion policies and the absence of such factors as single-sex wards, locked wards and nurses in uniform. However, he also speculates as to 'whether these hospitals rely on chemical restraint; have higher nurse/patient ratios; higher injury rates; more absenteeism without leave; and more referrals to, and fewer admissions from, special hospitals and secure units . . . ' (Leopoldt, 1985). As is the case when attempting to build theory on complex issues, the article very interestingly poses more questions than answers.

This brings us to the point at which some assumptions must be made. We have to assume that when a non-seclusion policy is operated, physical restraints and medication are not increased as a consequence. This is assumed on the basis that both physical and chemical restraints are as unacceptable as seclusion, if not more so. Consideration is now focused upon such factors as the levels of aggression, injuries sustained, staff stress, turnover and absenteeism, that may arise when non-seclusion policies are implemented.

In an excellent article on the evaluation of a non-seclusion policy, Kingdon and Bakewell (1988) studied observation as a replacement for seclusion over a 2-year period. Their study was carried out in a semirural health district of Nottinghamshire in which is also located a special hospital. The management of disturbed patients was based on three differing levels of nursing observation: special, in which one nurse closely shadows a specific patient; close, where a nurse knows the specific whereabouts of a designated patient at all times; and general, where only the general whereabouts of a patient is known at any one time.

Data were collected from a number of sources, which included community agencies such as the Prison Medical Officer, the Regional Secure Unit (RSU), the Probation Service, the Police and local community groups. Effects on staff were measured, as were medication levels and admission and discharge rates.

They reported that only two patients had to be transferred from the ward to a locked ward in another district, which was due to high levels of aggression putting staff and patients at too much risk. Both patients subsequently returned and were ultimately discharged following treatment. They also reported that there were no transfers necessary to either a special hospital or an RSU during the study period. There was also no transfer from the special hospital to the ward during the same period, despite the relatively higher number of patients from that district admitted into the special hospital. However, this is probably more to do with the transfer policy of the special hospital, rather than the non-seclusion policy.

Similarly, there was no evidence in the study to suggest that there were more psychiatric referrals to the hospital wing of the local prison rather than the ward on which the study was based. On contact, the Prison Medical Officer was of the opinion that he had not declined to refer to the ward because of levels of actual or potential aggression.

Kingdon and Bakewell (1988) went on to detail the actual number and types of violent incidents that occurred during their study, and announced that property damage was the target on three occasions, other patients were attacked on five occasions, and staff members assaulted on 42 occasions. Despite the fact that they provided no figures for comparison between seclusion policy and non-seclusion policy, they did report that they considered the number of violent incidents as being low over the 2-year period. By the same token, they reported on medication levels for their study group but failed to provide comparative data for those being medicated in an area that used seclusion.

Finally, they related how, despite the anticipated staffing requirements being assessed as high, difficulties in recruitment led to a ratio below what was considered normal. They did not anticipate any greater difficulties had the staffing levels been as expected. Interestingly, they touch on what must be a major determinant in any quest to adopt a non-seclusion policy: 'staff morale, however, we do believe to be fundamentally important, supported by prompt and unambivalent responses from senior nursing and medical staff' (Kingdon and Bakewell, 1988).

Clearly, a non-seclusion policy, if attempted realistically and appropriately, must deal with the issue of assaultative behaviour. Despite the many interventions that can be applied to reduce, assess, divert or manage violence, it would be nonsensical to claim to have eradicated it in all circumstances. Violent incidents in many care settings remain unacceptably high, and the under-reporting of these incidents is well documented in the literature (Lion, Snyder and Merrill, 1981). Often in these settings violent outbursts are expected and are seen as part of the job. This can lead to serious problems of machoism and images of 'toughness', as discussed in Chapter 6. It is also fraught with clinical dangers. In one hospital a severely disturbed autistic teenager made, on average, six attacks per day, which the staff accepted and considered routine. As the attacks became 'normal', so did the bites, scratches and bruises the staff received, which led them to cease recording them. After several weeks the psychiatrist concerned noted that the number of attacks reported had reduced considerably, and ultimately stopped altogether. Claiming a treatment success, he referred the patient for discharge – unsuccessfully.

The need to provide appropriate support mechanisms for those on the receiving end of such violence is both a multidisciplinary imperative and a nursing management responsibility. Without an assessment of the consequences of a non-seclusion policy, and a resolution of each of the problems that may be encountered, there appears little moral justification for putting other patients and staff at more risk than they need to be. The problem of assessment was summed up by Kingdon and Bakewell, (1988): 'it is certainly possible that such a policy can only be pursued in an 'average' area such as Bassetlaw, and that inner cities . . . , with their more serious social problems, would have greater difficulties'. This leads to the considerations of a non-seclusion policy.

CONSIDERATIONS

Any non-seclusion policy requires contextualizing in terms of the type of establishment in which it will be used, and identifying what could be interpreted as the underlying philosophies.

The type of patient catered for is central to an analysis of the feasibility of reducing seclusion rates and establishing non-seclusion, as is describing the practice philosophy of the units concerned. For example, Wells' (1972) study, in which he reports a 4% seclusion rate, is referring to a university medical centre psychiatric floor with a 12-bedded locked area. The unit has 22 beds in total and is well staffed with ' . . . three first-year psychiatric residents, a rotating intern, a third-year chief resident, three medical students, an activities coordinator, plus a psychiatric social work aide . . . ', who are all supervised by a clinical director. They also boast a head nurse and a nurse clinician accompanied by five or six nurses on day shifts. This teaching unit has small numbers of general psychiatric patients, with considerable staff input. They adopt a multidisciplinary approach and work along individualized care plan lines.

Soloff (1978) also reported low seclusion rates from his study in a military teaching hospital, which employed milieu therapy, group therapy and patient-involved management, and had a multidisciplinary team approach with a high staff–patient ratio. Although his study focused on the use of restraints, which were used in the unit under investigation, the seclusion rates reported were relatively low.

Mattson and Sacks' (1978) study also reported relatively low seclusion rates of 7.2%. However, their study was set in a private voluntary psychiatric division in a general hospital. They report that the unit was heavily staffed and served as a teaching unit. It seems fair to suggest that in such a facility patients would be expected to be to some degree amenable to treatment, and therefore compliant. Perhaps the surprising thing is that seclusion is used for voluntary patients in the first place.

We saw earlier that Wadeson and Carpenter (1976) reported the highest seclusion rates (66%) in their study based on an NIMH clinical research unit for acute schizophrenic patients. However, they also reported that they used medication very sparingly, and not at all while the patients were being assessed. To manage such acute patients without the use of drugs is certainly a very challenging approach indeed. It is not too surprising that the seclusion rates were so high during what must have been periods of extremely florid psychotic phenomena.

In the debate regarding the balance between seclusion, restraints and medication, there is a suggestion that if seclusion is eliminated then levels of medication and/or restraints would be increased to maintain control. Those that do not have a seclusion facility and claim that medication levels have not increased would contradict Wadeson and Carpenter's findings, which clearly links high use of seclusion with low medication.

Later studies are also based on the general psychiatric patient, for example, Morrison, P. (1990) in his study, stated: 'the unit was made up of five wards in a newly constructed psychiatric block in a large general hospital; two wards in a traditional psychiatric hospital; and a house in the community which was converted into an admission unit'.

The different types of patient groups, although rarely discussed at length, range from private psychiatric patients to the compulsorily detained, and as extremely violent and criminal patients gravitate to secure units and special hospitals this must be a consideration in developing a non-seclusion policy.

The development of a non-seclusion policy is a laudable enterprise, but only if great care is taken to protect all concerned. It is morally indefensible to claim the elimination of the use of seclusion if others are thereby caused harm.

Part of the problem, of course, is that since dangerousness and violence have been brought under the influence of psychiatry there is a need to apply the medical model to them. This includes diagnosis (assessment), treatment (intervention) and prognosis (prediction), and it is fair to conclude that notable authors on these topics are, as yet, far from being accurate or effective in any of the component parts of the model in relation to dangerousness and violence.

This is one reason why, whenever any controls are removed from the options available to nurses who deal with violence, anxiety is understandably raised. Such removal forces nurses to review their own, and others', capabilities, and to assess the viability of alternatives. This can be a good thing, but when these alternatives fail and the patient becomes assaultative it can be an immensely fear-inducing work environment, which is unhealthy for all. The feelings of inevitability, impotence and foreboding can produce high levels of stress for both staff and other patients.

There are many issues within this framework, which will be briefly pointed out. The first is the role of hospital managers in providing a healthy and safe working environment. This was outlined in Chapter 5. Secondly, it is often left to others, who may not be working in direct patient contact, to produce ideological statements, which are bound up with policy, often unrealistic, and provide the environment for the emergence of bad practice. Thirdly, without some controlling social mechanism aberrant behaviour tends to get worse, not better. When this occurs, nursing practice which has been made sterile produces staff who will withdraw from patient contact. This leads to less effective therapy and exacerbates mental and behavioural conditions. At one unit, whose management boasts a non-seclusion policy, ward nursing staff told of a clique of psychopathically disordered patients who dominated the ward, roaming from area to area, threatening and terrorizing other patients and staff. The nursing staff claimed that very little support came from those staff off the ward, and they felt helpless to intervene. These nursing staff, in fear for their own safety, were forced to develop illicit methods of control which were hidden from management. Meanwhile, the management flattered themselves on the use of 'new' techniques in managing disturbed behaviours. Little did they know (or perhaps they ignored) that behind the scenes the methods employed were as primitive as ever. Worse, they were hidden and open to abuse. This, it must be emphasized, is most definitely *not* a non-seclusion policy: it is a non-therapeutic, unhealthy and unacceptable state of affairs.

The fourth issue, however, must be to work towards the realistic and safe development of alternative methods of managing dangerous and violent behaviours. This must be done within the schema of reducing seclusion to an absolute minimum and providing a support framework for the safety of those in the clinical areas, with the ultimate goal of eradicating the use of seclusion altogether.

ALTERNATIVES

We now accept that the use of seclusion has no therapeutic benefit, and that all that it offers could be given without the use of a locked door: time alone could be offered without denying egress; respite from the intensity of the ward environment could be arranged without denying egress; and so on. We also accept that there is no role for the use of seclusion as a punishment, although we recognize that there may be a need (American

Psychiatric Association, 1984), to provide a controlling mechanism, in the form of sanctions, in any institution that manages human beings. Therefore, we are left with the use of seclusion merely as a means of containment, for the protection of others not the patient himself. Self-injurious behaviours and threatened or attempted suicide should be managed in a different manner, with staff in attendance. The containment principle (Gutheil, 1978; Mason, 1993a) is based on the reduction of risk to others. As has been pointed out (Chapter 4), although some authors have attempted to couch this in psychodynamic terms (Hodgkinson, 1985) it appears to us that this is merely an attempt to legitimize seclusion use as a 'medicalized' intervention, thus giving it 'professional' credibility. It may be the case that the 'containment of personal relationships' is inadequate, or that the patient may need an environment in which their 'fragile ego boundaries may be restored', but is seclusion really the appropriate method? Honesty compels us to admit that the majority of nurses using seclusion do so not because of the psychological implications but because violence must be contained to protect staff and other patients.

Turning now to alternatives to seclusion, which is the pivot on which the development of a non-seclusion policy must rotate, we must first understand what does and does not constitute an alternative. Phrases such as 'we do not use seclusion, we use an alternative', or 'seclusion is an outmoded intervention', or 'we adopt more modern alternatives' are very popular in many psychiatric disciplines. However, there is seldom any evidence given of a true alternative, but merely reworked tried and tested (and failed) precursors to the use of seclusion. This is not new, as Gair (1980) stated: 'lesser limits than seclusion are not truly alternatives – they are precursors. When they suffice there is no need for seclusion'.

If we accept that seclusion is not therapeutic, and should not be used for punitive reasons, nor for the protection of the patient, but only to prevent significant injury to others, then clearly this makes seclusion an emergency measure in response to extremes of violence. With this in mind, it is difficult to see how the suggested alternatives can be appropriate. If a patient is in the throes of combat, is it appropriate to play a relaxation tape? If a patient is in the process of assault, is a diversionary strategy the first 'alternative' to restraint? Quite clearly, no. Why not try restraint by holding? There is no reason why not, if that is enough.

To reiterate, precursors are not truly 'alternatives', they are those diverse approaches, strategies and interventions that are vigorously attempted *before* restraint and/or seclusion is deemed necessary. This is a crucial point to understand in any realistic attempt to develop a non-seclusion policy. The use of these precursors is essential in fostering such a policy. While it is recognized that many staff possess, and exercise, a high degree of clinical skill and expertise, it is also important to constantly review personal abilities and identify areas for development and expansion in the area of precursors.

PRECURSORS

The grouping of some precursors under the various headings below is quite arbitrary, and is done merely for the sake of structure. Many of the precursors will be very obvious to some but not to others. Also, many are the very basic skills of psychiatric nursing, which readers will readily recognize.

Staffing precursors to a non-seclusion policy

The relationship between staffing and violence (and seclusion) on the ward is complex. There are studies that suggest that high seclusion rates correlate with higher staffing levels, while other studies report a similar correlation between high seclusion rates and low staffing levels. There is also the issue of the appropriate gender mix of the nursing staff on duty, as well as their individual level of skills. Getting the right balance between these factors relies on such things as good management skills, which incorporate the ability to accurately gauge the competence and weaknesses of staff, to audit the varying needs of both staff and patients, and the expertise to appropriately assess the resource implications.

However, an increase in resources is not always necessary to develop some of the precursors, although it is accepted that more resources may be beneficial. Often, if staff morale is high, if management have organized the hospital to instil, maintain and encourage enthusiasm and motivation, and the staff are professionally inspired, then such individual factors as initiative, resourcefulness and the ability to think laterally can significantly reduce violence and/or seclusion. Too many staff can be as bad as too few staff, but in relating staffing to the use of seclusion, Craig, Ray and Hix (1989) reported that 'our suspicion that staffing patterns had a strong impact on this issue was verified'.

Environmental precursors to a non-seclusion policy

It is well understood that the majority of people do respond in one way or another to their environment. From the very simplest aspects, such as brightness of decor and pleasant furnishings, to more complex and personalized aspects, such as freedom of movement and the provision of personal space, all can have profound effects on a person's mental state. Wherever possible, access to open space, the reduction of overcrowding and the provision of quiet rooms can reduce the tensions and friction that lead to violence and seclusion.

The ward structure and design – almost always out of the hands of those who work and live in it – is crucial in providing a stimulating, but not overbearing, environment. This is especially true of many of the locked wards, in which patients may be confined for long periods of the day. Safe access to amenities such as telephones, hot water etc., within the ward is extremely significant for those restricted within its boundaries and it is appreciated that these can be problematic and abused by patients; however, with ingenuity, inventiveness and creativity most problems can be overcome (Greenblatt, 1980).

The patient mix is often overlooked as a precursor to many problems on the ward. Sometimes those patients who are more capable can dominate those less able, and an awareness of intimidation and abuse is important.

We accept that with some, particularly the severely mentally impaired, their appreciation of pleasant surroundings is not always obvious, and often does not, or cannot, alter disturbing behaviours, such as urinating on the ward and smearing faeces. However, imaginative and inspired nursing can often help prevent deterioration to the harsh, bleak conditions to be seen in certain very demanding care settings. The severe condition of some patients is no excuse for not trying.

Clinical precursors to a non-seclusion policy

Arguably the most important factor in reducing the levels of violence and/or seclusion on the wards is staff skills. Nurses all have areas in which they excel, and all are different. The important point is that learned skills require constant revision, updating and expanding upon if they are to be effective in providing a quality service.

There are, of course, many psychiatric skills and techniques above and beyond those mentioned here, and many people will feel that they exercise these on a daily basis. However, a review of personal skills may remind us of other approaches that have lain dormant.

Irwin (1987) discusses the role of milieu therapy and its constructs in reducing seclusion. Milieu therapy is a popular phrase to use when we cannot think of any other reason why a patient is admitted to the ward, and other interventions appear useless. Yet, on examining some of the constructs of milieu therapy, not only is it possible to appreciate its role, but by focusing on its constituent parts we are able to enhance and develop each construct much more effectively. For example, once stated, some of the constructs appear very familiar, such as processing, negotiating, slow-down periods, verbal de-escalation, relaxation techniques, self-soothing skills, alternate coping and stress-reducing strategies (Irwin, 1987). These are terms that cover aspects of psychiatric nursing with which we are familiar, and yet, if applied objectively, with the theoretical constructs in mind, the entire process becomes much more systematic. Through this reflective approach, developments can occur via the constant feedback and evaluation that lead to variations being attempted. Within the theoretical application of milieu therapy we may also include limit setting, in which boundaries are defined by negotiation beyond which sanctions will be applied. Avoidance of power struggles between staff and patients, staff and staff, and patient and patient, is vitally important in reducing the use of seclusion (Gair, 1980). Interactive encounters are the cornerstone of relationship formation. Unfortunately, if these encounters incorporate an element of domination, based on a hierarchical structure of power relations, then positions become entrenched and attitudes become intransigent. This can lead to stagnation, which must be avoided if progress is to be made.

An understanding of group and ward dynamics is also central in operating a non-threatening environment. Inexperienced nursing staff and managers can become inextricably embroiled in cleverly constructed power struggles set up by very adept personality-disordered people. Gentilin (1987) was extremely aware of this, and emphasized extreme caution, awareness, and avoidance of levelling, scapegoatism, transference diffusion, clique formation and peer-age caricaturing.

Van Rybroek *et al.* (1987) focused on the awareness and interruption of the aggression cycle, which involves the following sequence: aggression, seclusion, fear, social distancing, return of aggressive behaviour and seclusion. This cycle is self-perpetuating, and is made worse by the impotence of staff to intervene and break the cycle, especially when there is a lack of cohesiveness on the ward and little ability to take a step back and try alternatives.

In developing a non-seclusion policy there are, of course, many approaches using precursors to prevent the deterioration towards the use of seclusion. Familiar ones include one-to-one observations, appropriate use of PRN medication, diversional therapy, behaviour modification techniques, peer-group social exclusion and providing opportunities to be alone. There are many more.

Should the situation deteriorate to what may be considered an impending disturbance, then it is still important to remain calm. Understanding the various factors that may contribute to the appropriate assessment of this situation can raise fresh initiatives, depending on each individual situation, and focuses a unique approach to each set of circumstances. Violence is a fear-inducing behaviour, the response to which is the production of adrenalin. This is nature's way to prepare a person for 'fight or flight'. As flight is not often an option for those present at a violent disturbance, it is understandable that 'fight' becomes the expected option, and nature provides the optimum state for the application of maximum strength. This can clearly lead to automatic excessive force. To override this, psychiatric nurses are taught to develop skills and techniques, not only to prevent violence, but also for the calm objective assessment of violent outbursts and the effective appropriate responses to them.

One of these responses is distance rationalizing. This is similar to a hostage situation, in which a dialogue is initiated as early as possible, from a distance, with the intention of engaging, and thus distracting, the disturbed person from carrying out the intended violence.

Education and development of clinical practice

Education, both formal and informal, is central to the seclusion debate: sensible constructive criticism can provide the basis for innovation and change, whereas blind, blinkered ideology can prevent any hope of development. As this is covered in Chapter 8, only brief mention will be made here.

There is no easy way out of the seclusion polemic. The realistic establishment of a non-seclusion policy is an objective which requires careful management of the highest calibre. Even the reduction of seclusion rates is no simple manner, as Greenblatt (1980) pointed out: 'required for this to happen were the long hours of discussion and teaching of staff. . . . '

This is, once again, one aspect which requires a stretching of both mind and imagination. Davidson, Hemingway and Wysoki, (1984) argued that very basic instructions and feedback to staff could significantly reduce seclusion rates. Ishiyama and Hewitt (1966) suggested that staff on induction and in-service programmes should experience seclusion themselves, for a short length of time. Other educative approaches included an incident debriefing exercise for all concerned following each and every seclusion, and the setting up of a Seclusion Advisory Team to assess seclusions and involve themselves in post-seclusion discussions (Macdonald, 1989). Without doubt, seclusion should be part of the nursing curriculum, at the very least as one of a number of contentious issues.

Multidisciplinary involvement

It must be remembered that seclusion use and its reduction is of multidisciplinary concern. Although it is accepted that the nurses have the greatest 'hands-on' responsibility, each member of the team should contribute in assessment, implementation and evaluation of their role. Each member should take responsibility for the failure to prevent seclusion being initiated, and should strive to develop realistic opportunities for alternative management.

Nurse–patient relationship

Clinical nurses stand in a unique position regarding patient care, as they operate in close proximity to the patient for the greatest length of time. The development of a professional therapeutic nurse–patient relationship is vital to the effectiveness of care delivery. The importance of such concepts as primary nursing and key worker cannot be over stressed, and the construction of care plans should be undertaken rigorously and incisively, rather than repetitively and meaninglessly. 'Little did they (the staff) realize the power of attitudes, fears, and prejudices they might hold towards those in their charge to induce either apprehension and suspiciousness on the one hand, or trust and comfort on the other' (Greenblatt, 1980).

NON-SECLUSION THEORY AND RESOURCES

The authors hope they have been down to earth, pragmatic and realistic in relation to the development of a non-seclusion policy, and not nonsensical, ideological and platitudinal in the construction of yet another nursing facade by claiming the high moral ground. In going some way towards constructing a theory of a non-seclusion policy, we have based it on the age-old need to protect, the type of patient group catered for, the difference between alternatives and precursors, and the necessity of developing these and other precursors if advancement is to be forthcoming.

We have not shied away from the many problems that may be encountered, both the visible official ones and the unofficial hidden ones, and would point out the necessity of overcoming these problems with inventiveness, lateral thinking and imagination.

Although with some initiatives in developing a non-seclusion policy extra resources are not strictly necessary, it is vital to understand that in other cases extra resources must be made available if the policy is to succeed. It would be unjust to expect staff and patients to put themselves at risk to satisfy a management objective. Resources include management skills, expertise, understanding, support and safety, as well as finance for training, ward design and decor, staffing etc.

Managers, particularly nursing managers, must provide a

realistic support framework for those staff who take calculated risks with alternative management of disturbed behaviour. This support framework should be strengthened considerably when things go wrong, as they will from time to time. It is inappropriate and a sign of bad management merely to provide pressure to change and then punish the change agents when the risks have been taken and events have turned out negatively. Management overreaction smothers the motivation for change and reinforces the routine and ritual of traditional policies.

We began this chapter by indicating the four options available in dealing with the extremely aggressive patient, when all precursors have been tried and failed, when the patient becomes combatant and is in the throes of repeated attacks, namely: seclusion, restraint, medication and transferring the patient elsewhere. These are the only true alternatives to the use of seclusion, but can increasing restraints and medication justifiably be termed alternatives? It would appear that by increasing these equally distasteful mechanisms of control, they also have the potential to become part of the seclusion abuse.

8

Seclusion and nurse education

Ann Alty

Angold (1989) points out that very often practitioners are not trained to carry out seclusion or to understand the underlying principles of its use. Frequently, the topic is not discussed in nurse training or education.

CURRENT PREREGISTRATION EDUCATION ON SECLUSION

A small survey was carried out by one of the authors in order to ascertain what teaching takes place in current nurse curricula. Ten colleges of nursing were approached within one northern health region. Each college was asked to complete a questionnaire regarding their teaching on seclusion. There was a mixture of colleges represented, some continuing traditional courses and others with Project 2000 students completing their mental health branch experience. Of the ten colleges approached, eight responded by completing and returning their questionnaires. Of these, only two (one-quarter) taught anything about seclusion to preregistration nursing students and only one of these included seclusion as a named part of the curriculum. Seven colleges claimed to teach associated subjects which might be useful in implementing seclusion. These included aggression, rights issues, assertiveness, counselling, ethics, law and 'therapeutic approaches/techniques that may make seclusion less of an option'.

In response to being asked: 'Do you feel that seclusion is adequately addressed in preregistration education?', four out of six of those not teaching about seclusion answered 'No', with the other two declining to answer. One respondent claimed that

'Seclusion is no longer an issue' in support of not teaching seclusion. One respondent claimed that seclusion was not adequately addressed because of lack of knowledge by teaching staff. Another reason proffered by two of the respondents was that P2000 courses were too busy and too generalized to include teaching on seclusion. Of the colleges who did not teach about seclusion, one claimed that seclusion was not practised on the training wards and one was not sure if it was used. Yet because seclusion is not used on training wards it does not necessarily follow that the qualified nurse has no contact with seclusion practice at a later date.

Obviously, a brief pilot study is very limited in value as to the real picture; however, it does appear that there is no standard approach to teaching seclusion practice among nurse educators, and that some Health Authorities and Trusts within a small geographical area can have completely opposing views as to the value and importance of educating students about seclusion usage. Yet even in areas where seclusion is practised there is little, if any, education as to its implementation; one respondent even stated that it was the responsibility of ward nursing staff to teach about seclusion. For the majority of students and Registered Mental Nurses, therefore, it would appear that seclusion is carried out and learned by simply being involved and observing its implementation at ward level.

It is interesting to hear how nursing students prior to Project 2000 actually learned about seclusion. One registered staff nurse says:

'I remember vividly the first time I observed seclusion being used. As a first-year student on an acute ward I came on duty one morning to find the nurses acting secretively. I was instructed not to go down to the seclusion area as they did not want to disturb the patient who had been placed in there overnight as he had been extremely violent on admission. I helped the female patients to get dressed. The seclusion room was close to the female dormitory and I remember feeling extremely curious and not a little anxious about the fact that we had another human being locked away at such close quarters. It was terrifying really. At break time I was asked to help the staff nurse ensure that the patient had a drink and was toileted. I hovered near the doorway as the patient drank his tea and took his medication. He looked lost and his eyes seemed dazed. I remember how scruffy he looked. I asked once why he was there and was told that he had been extremely violent on admission. The tone of the reply ensured that I didn't ask any more questions! I was a student and didn't need to know the ins and outs of the decision making. The patient was discharged soon afterwards. I just remember that it was all very mysterious and strange but was afraid of looking stupid by asking questions. Instead, I adopted a bravado which I observed in the trained staff which appeared to me to be matter of fact and unquestioning about the reasons for it all.'

Another staff nurse who was interviewed about her seclusion experience responded thus:

I. Were you ever given any training or teaching about seclusion?
S.N. None whatsoever. I was given the seclusion policy to look at.
I. When did you first see seclusion being used?
S.N. On my first ward placement. I helped bundle someone away and I had no teaching at this stage either. It was more of an understanding that if someone was 'wild' and 'uncontrollable' they go into seclusion.
I. Have you ever found seclusion helpful?
S.N. As an RMN I used seclusion once to benefit a patient who found the ward was too stimulating – 'open seclusion' – my own experience enabled me to judge the appropriateness of this and how long to use it.

The above nurses are both practising staff nurses and neither have had any training or formal teaching about seclusion.

It appears from the above that nurse curricula have so far failed to address issues such as seclusion adequately. Indeed, it has been stated that 'The present system of nurse education is failing to meet the needs of a substantial number of learners' (Kendrick and Simpson, 1992). In a study of charge nurses working in psychiatric admission units, Cormack (1976) states: 'It can be said that the observed nurses were not carrying out a role which was equivalent or even similar to that which was prescribed by many of the contributors to contemporary nursing literature' (Cormack, 1976). Cormack felt that charge nurses were not equipped during training to take charge of wards or to perform to his 'prescribed role'.

It is, of course, easy to criticize outcomes without understanding the whole picture of practice. There are three main areas which seem prevalent in causing problems and flaws in nurse education concerning seclusion; these are nurse socialization factors, medicalization of nursing practice and bureaucratic obstacles to innovative practice.

NURSE SOCIALIZATION

It is felt that nurse socialization plays a major part in carrying out tasks and performing as a nurse. Nurse education has always been much more than enabling a student to carry out various tasks or to learn theories of nursing. The transition from student to nurse has been studied at great length by various people and has highlighted the fact that nurse education has much to do with socialization of nurses. Indeed, it has been pointed out that 'education is the master socialization process' (Simpson, 1979), which underlines the fact that nurses are actually learning more about the socialization of nurses than nursing theory when they enrol on various training or education courses. It has been pointed out that past nurse education has stifled innovation (Auld, 1992), and it appears that education is more effective as a means of socializing rather than having knowledge and understanding of a defined subject. Nursing is therefore not so much an educational qualification but a combination of educational understanding and socialization which results in practice. Unfortunately, the educational understanding and social norms will sometimes conflict. Powell (1982) points out that changes in education must also include already trained staff who work in psychiatric wards. In his study he found that trainees concentrated more on establishing relationships with ward staff rather than with the patients they were caring for. Subsequent behaviour was therefore defined by staff already on the ward in which they were nursing, rather than based on what they learned in the training school. Powell concludes: 'Change in psychiatric nursing is unlikely to occur in the absence of informed role models' (Powell, 1982). In examining the subject of seclusion it is paramount that this socialization process is addressed. As we have already pointed out, learning the practice and procedure of seclusion happens at ward level and never in the classroom. It follows, therefore, as Powell discovered, that the practice will inevitably demonstrate the values and understanding of the environment in which it is carried out, rather than research-based theory and practice. Given that ward environments also differ it is not surprising that Angold (1989) discovered that the practice of seclusion differs greatly from unit to unit and from health authority to health authority, and this is supported in the brief pilot study described above.

MEDICALIZATION OF PSYCHIATRIC NURSING PRACTICE

Lancaster (1982) states: 'Perhaps one of the greatest impediments to the delivery of health care services has been the way in which providers have traditionally conceptualized the recipients of their care. The recipients of health care have generally been referred to as patients which connotes a passive, dependent role'. Lancaster then states that change is of paramount importance, 'Not only in nursing but also in the entire health care system' (Lancaster, 1982). This is possibly largely due to the fact that psychiatric nursing has relied heavily on the medicalization of mental health for its knowledge base. The authors recall only too well the lectures received during training. Psychiatric lectures were often given by medical staff as a whole set of signs and symptoms, which encouraged labelling and complacency in attempting to understand patients as unique individuals. The 'hands on' treatment afforded patients following such lectures and training was predictably widely off the mark in enabling us to empathize and listen to the patients in our care. This lack of expertise felt uncomfortable for a time, but was viewed as inexperience by those around us. Experienced nurses knew how not to get involved with their patients, and this was considered (by the profession) to be the trademark of good nursing over the past few decades.

Gender also plays a part in maintaining this medical dominance within psychiatric nursing. Nursing traditionally takes the form of training individuals, usually women, to carry out tasks and assist doctors (usually men) in the care of the patient. Thus nursing is seen as a role which lends itself to unquestioning obedience to the medical staff, and it has been argued that it is inextricably intertwined with the subordination of women. This continues to be reflected within psychiatric nursing, even when more men are traditionally employed within mental health. Cormack (1976) observed interactions between nurses and doctors in his study and described the nurse's role as definitely subservient to the medical staff (Cormack, 1976). Some would argue that not much has changed in present practice (Salvage, 1985; Savage, 1987; Clay 1987). It was pointed out that in 1980 the most senior positions in nursing were almost exactly equally divided between men and women, with female posts accounting for just over 50% of those studied. This seems fairly equal and fair at first glance, until one realizes that only 10% of the total nursing population was male at the time (Salvage, 1985). Not only do men seem to dominate the senior positions within the profession, which adds to the subordination of women argument, but nurses are still considered to be subservient to medical staff as a profession, possibly for similar reasons; female nurses do make up the majority of nursing positions at less senior levels, which means that in general interaction with medical staff on the ward concerning patient care it is usually women who represent the profession. This means that the nursing staff have to negotiate on behalf of their patients and put forward nursing opinion in a way which fits in with the paternalistic doctor–nurse relationship. For example, Price (1985) points out that during the consultants' ward round the nurse may 'indicate certain nursing proposals but these must be presented in such a way that the doctor can adopt them without losing face'. Indeed, one of the authors approached an ethics committee in order to carry out research at a hospital, and was told that nurses could not carry out research without written permission from the consultant. No mention was made, however, of nurses being approached when medical staff proposed their own research.

The medical model has depersonalized patients and denied nurses the holistic approach to care, which values patients as individuals, not passive recipients of other people's decisions, nor as labelled illnesses which ignore or suppress the uniqueness of individuals and their ongoing development. This reductionist model of care has been sharply criticized: 'For nurses, the slavish pursuit of the reductionist medical model has resulted in the attrition of caring – the essence of our practice' (Farmer, 1993).

However, changes in the appreciation of such effects on practice are becoming more readily heard (Webster, 1990).

It has been pointed out that 'The out-dated curriculum is viewed often as a watered-down medical approach' (Kendrick and Simpson, 1992), and Farmer (1993) holds that education has been the dominant mechanism whereby nurses continue to be oppressed within their role. She maintains that a carefully controlled education system prevents nurses disrupting the status quo as they gradually internalize the values and beliefs of their organization, in the unfounded hope that nurses (the oppressed group) will eventually wield their own power within the organization. Unfortunately, this reductionist approach to health creates tension which, Farmer claims, leads to intergroup conflict and neglect of the people nurses are purported to be caring for: the patients.

In a study of nurse education among general nurses Gallego (1983) states: 'The future of evaluation in nursing may rest in its progress from being a technological process into becoming more of a social process. Perhaps only then nurse education may lead in fields where it has always followed'.

This comparatively early study demonstrated the need for nurses to assert themselves as practitioners in their own right, rather than as eclectic workers who could only glean from other fields rather than create their own knowledge base and practice. This reflected the continuing shift throughout the 1960s and 1970s, whereby nurses began to develop their own theoretical constructs and models to improve patient care. These attempts have been criticized for being somewhat naive (and indeed, some early studies did reflect this criticism when it came to analysis), and strong arguments have arisen as to whether nursing should be considered to be a profession in its own right (Salvage, 1988). Despite this debate, however, nursing does appear to be developing into a more organized framework which allows for innovation and development along more original constructs. To do this, nurses have moved away from the concept of nurses as handmaidens and begun to develop their own understanding of the patients in their care.

NURSING BUREAUCRACY AND SECLUSION

A further complication in examining the issues surrounding seclusion within nurse education is the difficulties that students experience working within a bureaucratic organization. It has been pointed out that, 'The structure of the nursing profession remains authoritarian, and this makes free expression of opinion almost impossible' (Robb, 1967). Although this criticism was made in the 1960s, before major restructuring took place, experience has shown that there remains a large element of this authoritative structure to impede any outspoken views being expressed.

Negotiating this nursing bureaucracy is only one element of political involvement, and it has long been recognized that politically active nursing is frowned upon by the nursing establishment. In fact, it has been said that 'Nursing is perhaps the most unassertive profession in the UK' (Clay, 1987). This gives managers and organizations immense power, and can hinder any change (good or bad) which is attempted by an individual or group of individuals. Nurses are encouraged to be politically benign and to fall in with whatever the establishment thinks best, whether that establishment be the health authority or their own nursing management. Nurses are actively discouraged from engaging in political discourse, and it has been argued that because of this nurse training has 'failed to permit the nursing system to develop and meet the changing needs of society' (White, 1985). Indeed, in her book on political issues in nursing, White identifies three main interest groups within nursing which all vie for power within the greater organization of health care. These are the managers, the specialists (or professionalists) and the generalists. As we consider these interest groups we may identify with the characteristics observed below. The generalists might be considered to be the 'shop-floor' workers, consisting largely of unskilled or semiskilled workers. These seem to be the greatest in number and have interests in union negotiating power. They also believe that nursing does not require academic or higher qualifications.

The specialists are those nurses who feel that education is vital in their practice and seek to further their career and practice by focusing on one or more areas in great depth, thus becoming experts. Specialists are not so much concerned with financial gain, only in perfecting their skills and affording their patients the best care available. Specialists prefer to work alone, without constant supervision and consequently 'tend to challenge the status quo of a hierarchical structure' (White, 1985). This would support the view that Farmer described, and is discussed in the preceding section. These specialists do not internalize the values and beliefs of the hierarchical system which is so important in maintaining the power structures and status quo of an organization. This is therefore perceived as very threatening by those who believe that unquestioning compliance is the only way to gain the most out of a career in nursing.

Nurse managers are regarded as people who, of necessity, leave their values of practice behind once they enter the management milieu. They quickly learn to talk in 'management language' and often move into management by accident rather than design. Managers seem to be threatened very much by the specialists, as the specialists do not value power and prestige over personal development and expertise in caring. White goes on to point out that it is not surprising that conflict occurs between these three groups, because 'Each has its own needs and goals: the generalists seek for material rewards and a functional status in the nursing system; the specialists seek for professional authority and accountability; the managers seek for control' (White, 1985).

If the above is considered with regard to seclusion, it can be seen that there would be great difficulty in attempting to make changes within nursing practice. The generalists would want to continue to practice as they have always done. Because the generalist works well within a system and is more interested in material reward or professional status, he would not wish to consider making any independent approach to studying seclusion practice. Any specialists who attempt to bring about changes must be able to negotiate the power control of the managers and the apparent complacency of the generalists. The managers, however, by the nature of their responsibilities, tend to become more policy- than practice-orientated, so that political pressures become paramount in any decision-making strategies. Should any one of these groups desire to move towards changing practice and acknowledging new authority, the status quo of the establishment would become extremely insecure and feel subjectively threatened in the short term. No-one likes to be placed in such a vulnerable position and the interaction between these three nursing groups becomes fraught with mistrust.

In 1981, a social audit report highlighted the plight of those students who attempted to act on behalf of their patients against cruelty and neglect (Beardshaw, 1981). The students met with extremely difficult social and bureaucratic opposition as they attempted to defend the patients in their care. Many of the students left training or did not practise for very long once they had completed their course. 'Whistleblowing', as this kind of professional conflict has come to be known, is very difficult and fraught with emotive issues. Bringing the practice of seclusion into nursing curricula will undoubtedly lead to such conflict.

Other, more recent, cases highlight the difficulties encountered when the nurse attempts to call attention to issues which the establishment prefers to deal with privately, if at all. The Department of Health has recently drawn up draft guidelines concerning whistleblowing within the NHS in an attempt to assist practitioners break through the difficulties brought about by bureaucracy and political opposition. The preparation of the document has largely been welcomed, but sharp criticism has ensued following the draft publication, not least by Mr Pink, the charge nurse who drew attention to the plight of his patients by first attempting to negotiate the proper channels and then contacting the press. He states that the guidelines change nothing, as they are open to subjective interpretation. He writes: 'The guidelines encapsulate what most nurses believe to be the accepted NHS credo: 'If you value your job, keep your head down, your eyes closed and your mouth tightly shut' ' (Pink, 1993). This opinion is valid concerning the difficulty in bringing about change within the organization; however, as we have already seen, the dynamics are far more complex than at first envisaged. Mr Pink's campaign resulted in his losing his position as charge nurse where he worked. He definitely appears to have disrupted the status quo among nurse management. While Mr Pink's campaign is laudable because it brings such difficulties as professional accountability and bureaucratic rigidity to the forefront of public awareness, it is tempered with a naivete which can be (and has been) exploited by the organizational structures within which it arose.

A more recent example of these difficulties was in 1992, when nursing students from St Bartholomew's College of Nursing and

Midwifery faced disciplinary action by their college following a letter which set out details of poor standards at two elderly care units. It was underlined that the students were not being disciplined for whistleblowing but for their insolence and manner in making the complaint. Thirty-one students were involved and had taken advice on how to bring the poor standards to the notice of managers. As the editorial of the *Nursing Standard* stated on 16 September 1992, 'Of course, nobody forewarned them that the wild card which would determine their survival was the subjective interpretation of politeness' (Casey, 1992). Eventually, the disciplinary action was dropped when the students compromised and apologized for any 'perceived' insolence in the letter. Legal difficulties were also highlighted in this case due to the fact that the UKCC were powerless to intervene, as the complainants were students and not registered nurses, even though Reg Pyne, the Assistant Registrar, Standards and Ethics for the UKCC, publicly stated that the students ought not to be punished (Naish, 1992). Mr Pyne stated that he felt the student nurses had acted properly. It seems unjust that student nurses are not protected by the UKCC code of conduct in the same way as registered practitioners, and calls have subsequently been made to reassess student nurses' legal standing. There has been extremely sharp criticism of nurses' hierarchical structure within the NHS following this case: 'This 'when you are grown up, you will understand' hierarchical hangover renders students disempowered to act until they have had three years' socialisation into health service compromises' (Naish, 1992). The obvious inferred conclusion here is that by the time the socialization has occurred over 3 years, the students would not wish to complain for fear of upsetting the status quo.

The stress and uncertainty of making such a complaint, even *en masse*, must surely continue to ensure that students think seriously before making any further attempts at blowing the whistle on poor standards, and much more so in the case of seclusion, as there is already much subjectivity about when secluding the patient can be considered to be a reflection of poor standards of care.

ADVOCACY AND SECLUSION

Recently, much has been made of the role of nurse advocates in providing patient care. Witts (1992) points out that advocacy ought to be seen as a major influence in quality of care. He also points out that he has been unable to discover advocacy included in nursing curricula and, of necessity cites American literature on educating nurses about advocacy.

It is felt, however, that advocacy is a nurse's role (Copp, 1986), yet it has been pointed out that, although nurses acting as patient advocates is not a recent development, it has been overshadowed by loyalty to medical practitioners (Becker, 1986). Advocacy is very difficult to define and is a complex practice. Various under-standings of what advocacy entails include nurses acting as 'intermediaries' (Jones, 1982) and 'educators' (Rendon *et al.*, 1986), as well as informing and supporting patients in their own decisions (Kohnke, 1980). However, others would disagree. For example, within psychiatry there have been recent developments in advocacy which actually state that nurses cannot be advocates at all, as they will still represent the system and socialization of a bureaucracy which is not in the best interest of patients. It has been pointed out that students are often the ones best able to build a rapport with patients, and can thus be better placed to advocate for them (Wagg and Yurick, 1983). Presumably, this view anticipates that the socialization which occurs as nurses develop will inhibit their advocacy skills.

It is argued that true advocates are those who have been in exactly the same position as the patient, i.e. other patients. A document provided by MIND for service users recommends approaching agencies other than health professionals to act as advocates. They stress that it is important that someone who knew the patient's values and beliefs before the illness be con-sulted, as they are better placed to act as advocates (MIND, undated). This is interesting, as it is true that nurses acting as advocates have only the knowledge they gain through a relation-ship based on interaction impaired by illness. Indeed, in a policy document published by MIND on user involvement, it is stated: 'Advocacy must be independent. A keyworker, as gateway to resources, cannot act as an advocate because of a conflict of interest' (MIND, 1991).

Having a nurse as advocate may, however, be effective, as she will have knowledge of how to negotiate the health care system to obtain the best care for the patient. She couples her professional knowledge with her knowledge of the patient, including his limitations of information, and makes efforts to provide a forum for the patient's needs to be met. However, as Witts (1992) points out, we do not always act independently within a system but will be influenced by that system and will sometimes experience conflict between what we know should be done and what organizational and social constraints allow.

Addressing such issues might be threatening to would-be advocates, and this is so in the case of seclusion. Those who object to or scrutinize aspects of care delivery are not comfortable people to work with, and this perceived threat may lead to understandable interdisciplinary and intradisciplinary tension. It is the belief of the authors, however, that this tension and the reasons for it must be addressed and appreciated before any real progress can be made in the academic understanding of seclusion practice.

There are definite problems, however, in endorsing advocacy, not least in the confusion that arises from the differing definitions and expectations: 'Ambiguity in the definition of the 'why' and 'how' of advocacy and the debate on whether nurses are suited to the role of advocate have left the nursing profession in confusion' (Sutor, 1993). Nonetheless, the needs of patients within seclusion will always need to be considered. Advocacy is one means whereby the patients' cases can be put forward, and even if the nurse is not herself acting as advocate, practitioners and managers should at least give other agencies who can act as independent advocates a hearing. This hearing ought not to be based on emotive issues and events which have made up the majority of opinions on the subject of seclusion, but must be research-based.

However, the difficulties encountered in establishing advocacy in practice are outlined by Stein (1993) who states: 'Advocates are only a suitable starting point when the health service is truly committed to changing and challenging its present systems of service delivery'.

As we have pointed out, there are great difficulties in establishing whether the health service is truly committed to changing delivery or simply wants to provide new policies in order to give the appearance of changing. To recommend that advocacy is a valuable starting point for implementing change is to ignore the greater difficulties in understanding what is encountered whenever advocacy is attempted. First must come the commitment from the service providers to begin to change health care provision, and to begin to challenge the restrictive frameworks encountered in its structure.

THE IMPACT OF PROJECT 2000 ON NURSE EDUCATION

In 1984 a DHSS report underlined the fact that nurses felt that their training was wholly inadequate for their experience of staffing on the wards. This report and other criticisms (White, 1985) ensured that nurse education was kept firmly on the political agenda. The bureaucracy, socialization and medically based task-oriented approach left nurses with a sense of ineptitude when dealing with real patients and staff on the wards. An RCN report called for major changes in nurse education and highlighted a fear of the unknown as a major obstacle to these necessary reforms (RCN, 1985). Many nurses who trained during the past three decades will recall the old adage, 'You don't start learning until you pass your exams' and experientially this was correct. Decision-making and management were taught, but only insofar as the organization deemed it necessary. Dealing with conflict and critical analysis was never highlighted as a means of equipping trained nurses on the wards. Students were regarded as 'an extra pair of hands' and even into the 1980s nurse training held no academic value with many universities or colleges of further education. However, the UKCC responded to this appalling lack of foresight of previous nurse educationalists by drawing together a plan now known as Project 2000 (UKCC, 1986).

Project 2000 aimed to address the difficult issues described above, and focused on the case for change 'on educational grounds, on service grounds and on grounds of recruitment and retention' (UKCC, 1986). The paper of 1986 proposed that nurses needed to provide care for a community, rather than simply hospital-based care, and that this responsibility ought to be reflected in nurse education. It aimed to bring nurse education into line with national higher education qualifications and to break down the idea that students needed to obtain most of their education at ward level as an 'extra pair of hands'. It also aimed to provide 'flexible practitioners who have the confidence and readiness for change' (UKCC, 1986), and who will be more able to deal with a changing society and unpredictable health behaviours and illnesses.

Some viewed the 1986 paper as a move towards achieving professional status for nurses. However, it has been pointed out that the new reforms ought to be 'viewed more fruitfully as a struggle for survival through the evolution of a new occupational model, rather than as a covert quest for traditional professional status' (Salvage, 1988). Salvage feels that full professional status for nursing can never be achieved.

Project 2000 has been cautiously welcomed by nurse educationalists. Its top-down approach in implementation has, however, been fraught with problems as people adjust to rapid change, but Project 2000 has not been just an isolated innovation, and needs to be seen as part of a whole new ethos of government planning and care based on the 'New Right' ideology which emphasizes holism and self-direction. Dependency is frowned upon as a quality and independence of thought and innovation have been encouraged within carefully guarded structures. At the time of writing this book there has been little feedback as to the success of Project 2000, and longitudinal studies have not yet been made or analysed in depth, but the changing attitudes towards the standards of training, particularly the practice of nursing students being given full student status in colleges of further education and universities, is being hailed as a breakthrough. It will be interesting to view the outcomes of these new measures within psychiatric care.

There have, however, been reports that there are still some resistive attitudes to these changes. For instance, Mike Lowry, a Senior Lecturer of Project 2000 students, reports that 'Students complained frequently of criticism from non-Project 2000 students and staff in clinical areas' (Lowry, 1992).

A study of non-Project 2000 students highlighted 'friction' and 'hardened attitudes' towards the proposals, which it was felt was more to do with ignorance of the facts than actual experience (Ford and Jones, 1992). The Project 2000 students themselves, however, are appreciative of this new approach to learning, which is felt to be more advantageous to professional learning (Blackburn, 1992; Chamberlain, 1992).

It will also be interesting to observe the effects of Project 2000 students arriving on a ward where the trained staff have no experience of the most recent developments in nurse education.

Project 2000 students are deemed to have great responsibility in bringing about this change of attitudes within the ward environment (Chamberlain, 1992). However, this could conceivably cause more division between education and practice, as students are no longer 'controlled' by the ward managers. Owen (1988) calls for established education institutions not to abdicate responsibility in placing this new breed of nurse in established nursing practice, and says: 'To put new practitioners into a hostile environment would invalidate the whole adventure' (Owen, 1988). It will be most interesting to observe whether any conflict between the differently trained practitioners is protracted into the 2000s, or even beyond, as yet another divisive influence on practice.

There have, however, been some cautionary voices as regards introducing Project 2000 into mental health nursing. Porter (1992) states strongly that 'As long as nurses are expected to play a custodial role in psychiatric institutions, their therapeutic concerns will tend to be compromised by their need to maintain order, no matter how sophisticated their training', and claims that Project 2000 will be problematic in implementation because of the fact that institutional care continues to be used in psychiatry. Thus there is a conflict of interests and approaches to care which is emphasized in the area of seclusion practice. It is conceivably difficult to attempt to control an individual, as in seclusion, and build up a therapeutic 'shared relationship' which has the patient's needs at heart when they are physically forced into a locked room 'for their own good'.

CHANGING SECLUSION PRACTICE

It was pointed out by a World Health Organisation committee that 'Effective leadership is a key factor in motivating people, bringing about change, and maintaining morale' (World Health Organisation, 1984). This is perhaps one aspect of bringing about change in seclusion practice from a management perspective. However, change can only really begin when circumstances and events are put clearly into context and appreciated. The areas addressed above are some attempt at highlighting the context in which seclusion practice is taught and practised. The authors have also sought to underline the political and educational context, which will undoubtedly cause difficulties and understandable problems when bringing about change. These areas will be discussed in greater depth in the next chapter. Unfortunately, a great problem in addressing the issue of seclusion and its practice is that, in examining the facts, there is understandable difficulty in apportioning blame and setting out a simple plan to address the situation. If it is felt that seclusion has been wrongly used, then who is to blame? The organization? Education? The managers? or the individual who happened to be there at the time of the enquiry and then is identified as a scapegoat for the remainder of the evidence? It is all too easy to reach simplistic, subjective conclusions. The individual may have acted wrongly, but if he has never been afforded another way of dealing with a problem and the social structures stifle innovative practice, then the individual who is disciplined is only representative of the whole, and the matter ought not to be dropped until each factor has been addressed. The fact that the Scope of Professional Practice (UKCC, 1992b) for nurses stipulates that nurses must be personally accountable for their practice will only serve to accentuate this position of 'victim blaming', rather than prevent it. Because of all these complications it is extremely difficult to know where to start addressing the problems perceived. Unfortunately, much damage may be done to good nursing practice when enquiries are carried out. It can become so easy to throw the baby out with the bathwater!

In a study of nursing the World Health Organisation points out that 'Nursing practice and education are governed by legislation that is often archaic, determined by persons from other disciplines, detrimental to the status of the nurse, and not in tune with the needs of society' (WHO, 1982). Seclusion is one such area which illustrates this viewpoint: socialization, medicalization and bureaucratic obstacles all impede innovation and questioning of the practice of seclusion. The introduction of Project 2000 is attempting to address these problems, but change is often slow and difficult, particularly in the wake of so much reorganization in the 1970s and 1980s within British psychiatric practice. However, change is beginning to occur and research-based practice is becoming more common. It is timely that nurses are reclaiming their valuable position within mental health as practitioners in their own right, without recourse to other influences that inhibit their attempts to meet the needs of the communities they serve.

9

Seclusion abuse

Ann Alty and Tom Mason

Seclusion continues to be used within mental health, and some would argue that it is an abuse of the individual (Pilette, 1978; Sallah, 1992). Yet just because the feelings associated with seclusion are negative this does not necessarily invalidate the practice. All medical and nursing interventions are vulnerable to abuse, as are all relationships which involve trust and power. Stover and Nightingale (1985) point out this unique relationship between the healing professions and those they care for: 'In view of the extraordinary diversity of human cultures, it is remarkable that we find evidence everywhere of respect for healers'. This respect can be abused in many ways, and an understanding of what occurs when abuse takes place will help in the exploration of seclusion practice and encourage self-awareness among practitioners.

DEFINING ABUSE

When carrying out a literature search on abuse and abusive contexts one is faced with a plethora of information about child sexual abuse, abuse of women and abuse within the family, but very little is given to abuse within other contexts. A small number of texts are concerned with torture and extreme cases of abuse, and these can be useful in understanding some of the dynamics, but seclusion does not readily fit into these contexts, as the abuse (if it is such) is more to do with general neglect and misunderstanding than with deliberate and systematic intention. Yet some of these texts can make uncomfortable reading for those who recognize that often those who carry out atrocities against human beings, such as those in labour camps and Russian psychiatric hospitals, firmly believe that the end justifies the means.

There are some general findings which can help carers to be aware of and assess whether they are abusing the trust placed in them by their patients or by society. A general definition of abuse may be used to consider whether seclusion abuse does actually take place. The following dictionary definition associates many words and phrases which might be classified as 'abuse':

'1. To use incorrectly or improperly; misuse.
2. To maltreat.
3. To speak insultingly or cruelly to.
4. Improper, incorrect or excessive use.
5. Maltreatment of a person, injury.
6. Insulting or coarse speech.
7. An evil, unjust or corrupt practice.'
    (Collins, 1982)

Careful examination of these definitions in relation to seclusion will highlight many areas which could cause concern, and correctly label certain seclusion interventions as abusive. It is the opinion of the authors that seclusion abuse can and does occur within both forensic and general psychiatric practice. Hospital inquiry reports support this view. Seclusion has been used incorrectly by some and associated with punishment rather than treatment. During seclusion patients have been insulted and nurses have described it as being used too much at times (Beardshaw, 1981; Chruszcz, 1992). Seclusion has also resulted in injury, and even death (Francis, 1985). However, we wish to underline that, although all seclusion is vulnerable to abuse, not all seclusion is abusive.

A glance at the above definition quickly highlights the subjectivity encountered in establishing whether abuse has occurred, and this is reflected throughout related literature. It is difficult, at this stage in nursing research, to ascertain whether it is an evil practice or even to define what evil practices are. It is extremely difficult to define when seclusion is correctly used and not an abusive intervention. Often abuse will occur over time, and will not be identified as such. There are many reasons for this.

ESTABLISHING ABUSE

It has been pointed out that 'One of the main reasons seclusion has such a poor image is not because of its use . . . but its misuse' (Brennan, 1991). However, while some evidence of seclusion abuse is obvious, it is extremely difficult to state categorically whether or not much of seclusion practice is abusive. The reasons for using seclusion appear to be extremely subjective and difficult to measure. We have already discussed the difficulty in ascertaining levels of dangerousness and predictability of violence. The fine line between paternalism and (abusive) authoritarianism will be examined in detail in the next chapter. In other words, whether or not a patient is viewed as potentially violent is often down to guesswork and opinion by practitioners. While the nurse will attempt to be as accurate as possible and use past experience to make these predictions, each situation is different and it is always difficult to state what might have happened had seclusion not been used.

The use of seclusion is inexplicably idiosyncratic (Angold, 1989). Some units use it regularly and some never use it at all. For example, in a survey of intensive care units in England, set up especially to nurse extremely disturbed patients, it was found that more than half had no facilities for seclusion, with the researchers being unable to ascertain why this was (Ford and Jones, 1992). If one intensive care unit did not seclude, does this mean that those who did were abusing the patients in their care? Some practitioners would argue that they were but there is no evidence to support this opinion.

Savage (1991) feels that all psychiatry is a form of abuse and creates victim blaming, which 'maintains the social conditions which produced the victims in the first place'. It has been pointed out that 'The nature of psychiatry is such that the potential for its improper use is greater than in any other field of medicine' (Bloch and Reddaway, 1977). The reasons for this are manyfold, but Bloch and Reddaway try to set them out, the main one being that psychiatry's boundaries are not clearly defined and there are few available assessment criteria for diagnosis and treatment. Additionally, they point out that the mentally ill 'are often used as scapegoats for society's fears', which leads to the development of conflicting loyalty in health care professionals between the patient in their care and the institution that pays their wages.

ASSESSMENT CRITERIA

Psychiatric classification has been strongly criticized as a means of creating stigmatization and social segregation for the mentally ill (Szasz, 1983). It has also been said that 'By promoting Descartian dualism psychiatric diagnosis also turns moral judgements into medical truths, shifts blame for problem behaviours from social structures and networks to the victim and . . . can and has been used for political control' (Savage, 1991).

It is simple for practitioners to 'label' patients with easily accessible and understandable terminology. For example, 'schizophrenic' conjures up pictures of behaviour and disease presentation in the minds of professionals which may pre-empt any further assessment in one-to-one interaction. Medical staff have long realized that this kind of labelling can be detrimental to the patient, and much is now made of avoiding such labels in psychiatric care. Unfortunately, these discarded illness labels have now been replaced by adopted behavioural labels, which appear to create the same cycle of assumptive practice. In the area of seclusion practice people are labelled as 'aggressive', 'suicidal', 'violent', 'settled', without such behaviour being objectively quantified. If a careful evaluation of past history is not made, a person might be described as aggressive when in fact only abusive language was used. Outlaw and Lowery (1992) point out that predictions about potential violence 'might be erroneous. Thus there is ample room for injustice to occur'. This information, passed between health practitioners either written or verbally, could well lead to interaction with the patient which is inappropriate, and could include unnecessary precautionary interventions such as seclusion. Unfortunately, psychiatric care is extremely vulnerable to this kind of individualistic interpretation, which in turn is open to abuse.

INSTITUTIONS AND IDEOLOGY

Patients who are secluded are always secluded within an institutional framework. They are never secluded in the community setting, but rather are removed to areas which are felt to be more capable of providing appropriate care. Other psychiatric interventions will occur at home or on an outpatient basis, but outpatients are never secluded. This severely limits the factors which the hospital nurse has available to make accurate assessments. A community nurse has ready contact with the patient's home and family, and will be able to gain a more accurate understanding of the patient's difficulties within his social, environmental and physical context. When a person becomes an inpatient, it distorts the picture available for accurate diagnosis and intervention. The patient will not be free to act as he would at home as he adjusts to this new environment, nor will the hospital nurse have available information from relatives or a GP who have known the patient for a longer period. The hospital nurse has no choice but to use the knowledge gained on the ward, thus basing decisions on factors different from the patient's usual sphere of relationships.

Because seclusion occurs in an institutional setting it is necessary to know a little about the underlying difficulties encountered within such settings. Many inquiries into patient abuse have occurred within huge institutional care facilities. Patterns of malpractice within psychiatric institutions are evident, and include incidents concerning abuse of patients' and hospital property, abuse of patients' money, abuse of time-keeping, poor standards of care and treatment, and assault or even manslaughter of patients (Beardshaw, 1981). Rarely are hospital inquiry reports concerned with only one of these issues: there is often overlap, and these abuses reflect what can happen when monitoring is poor and vulnerable people are placed in the care of a large institution. There are many reasons for this. Rarely do carers set out to deliberately and wilfully deprive patients or abuse them, but the dynamics of the institution and the ideology of society can and do permeate into the treatment offered. Racism is one such example of this, and it has been argued that psychiatry even plays a part in upholding racism in cultures, because 'The methodology of psychiatry as a discipline is so structured as to lay itself wide open to absorb current ideas in society about people, and incorporate them into its theory and practice. It is not naturally geared to provide a lead in breaking with an ideology that is dominant in society' (Fernando, 1988).

Moss (1988) points out that nurses have shared attitudes and beliefs which make them resistant to external influences. These patterns are reflected in certain attitudes and generalizations about the people in their care, as well as towards other professions within the multidisciplinary team. As nurses are most

frequently in contact with the patients within mental health settings, the patients become vulnerable to these attitudes. A visit
by a consultant once a week hardly equates with the 24-hour care
provided by the nursing staff. If nursing staff share a collective
approach to the patient, then the consultant's intervention, being
minimal, affords the least influence within general everyday
interactions. Moss points out: 'While nurses today claim to be
concerned with the whole patient, developing nurse–patient
relationships, and individualized patient care, there is considerable evidence to suggest that nurses deal with types of people,
types of behaviour and types of illness rather than individual
patients' (Moss, 1988). Moss concludes that nurses tend to anticipate attributes within patients rather than the actual attributes
of the individuals they care for. This is obviously going to cause
great problems in implementing seclusion, particularly given
that nurses within institutions are unlikely to be influenced by
other factors that community nurses have to encounter and consider when making analyses.

ROLE OF THE INDIVIDUAL

Each individual must assess the extent to which he or she has a
part to play in the abuse of seclusion. As described at the beginning of the chapter, it can be argued that being locked in a room
is abuse *per se* (Pilette, 1978; Sallah, 1992), and it can also be
argued that it is a level of abuse that can be morally justified in
preventing harm to others (Miller, 1992). However, as in many
nursing, medical and psychology practices, it is not the intervention itself that constitutes abuse but rather the individual
application of that intervention.

There are many questions we should ask ourselves when
involved in secluding patients, not least of all our attitude
towards the patient involved. It would seem obvious to state
that one's attitude towards seclusion is as important, if not more
important, than the actual practice itself, as this holds true for
all interactive treatment modalities. However, its significance is
often overlooked. The attitude towards seclusion can affect, to
varying degrees, the fear of or indifference to seclusion, the
effectiveness or otherwise of ongoing regimes and the lingering
memories of past seclusion experiences. Attitudes, however, are
notoriously difficult to quantify and may not even become trans-

lated into behaviour. In a pilot study aimed at quantifying therapeutic attitudes in mental health nursing, Rolfe (1990) discovered
that therapeutic attitudes were reduced the more experienced a
nurse became. In fact, Rolfe discovered that Registered General
Nurse students were more likely to exhibit empathy, genuineness
and respect towards their patients than either Registered Mental
Nurse students or qualified nurses. This study, however, is very
limited as a pilot study and the author readily points this out.
His findings were very interesting though, and pose questions
as to why less measurable skills are demonstrated the longer a
nurse has been in contact with patients.

It is accepted from studies concerning seclusion practice that
there is variance between staff views of seclusion and that of
patients, which is not so remarkable when one considers that the
former administer it and the latter receive it. We would expect
the same results from parents and children regarding 'bad-tasting
medicine'. The terms parents and children are chosen carefully,
as studies suggest that patients thought that nursing staff felt
powerful and in control when secluding patients (Tooke and
Brown, in press), and patients have reported that they felt humiliated and punished (Soliday, 1985). This discrepancy is further
complicated by an ever-wider divide between what patients
believe staff think of seclusion and what staff say their beliefs
are (Heyman, 1987). Certainly it would appear that there is a
distinct breakdown in communication between staff and patients
regarding seclusion, and it certainly raises the question of
whether it really matters what someone thinks. After all, if the
recipient perceives it as bad then clearly it is, relatively speaking.

Part of the abuse may involve staff believing seclusion to be
efficacious for the patient, but there is little evidence that this is
really the case. When staff are asked about their attitude to
seclusion as a safe and effective therapeutic tool, they tend
to report positively and unambiguously in support (Kilgalen,
1977; Plutchik *et al.*, 1978; Soloff and Turner, 1981; Soliday, 1985).
However, this must be contrasted with some considerable disquiet reported by staff in other studies regarding seclusion usage
(Fitzgerald and Long, 1973; Strutt *et al.*, 1980; Convertino, Pinto
and Fiesta, 1980; Campbell, Shepard and Falconer, 1982). Often,
being labelled as 'better' or 'settled' refers more to behaviour
than mental state, and can very easily be interpreted as a form
of social control. As Brown and Tooke (1992) have argued,

'Patients who reported feeling calm during seclusion often simultaneously described themselves as angry and depressed. Apparently, being 'calm' does not necessarily imply a sense of psychic wellbeing'.

The abuse of seclusion is not always seen in terms of extended durations, spartan conditions and overt mistreatment; often it is subtly transmitted, but received with a big impact. One would anticipate that the use of seclusion is usually as a direct consequence of violence. However, this is not the case, as can be seen from the literature. The high seclusion rates reported in response to actual or threatened violence (Soloff and Turner, 1981; Thompson, 1987) suggests that staff feel a sense of personal safety when the patient is secluded. However, this must be challenged by evidence in Lion, Snyder and Merrill's (1981) study that the majority of assaults on staff occurred when the patients were being restrained, often prior to secluding them. As pointed out in Chapter 4, there are strong suggestions that the use, frequency and duration of seclusion are closely related to the extent to which staff dignity has been offended (Binder, 1979; Soloff, 1987). Such affronts can range from assault to non-compliance, and in many cases the use of seclusion is rationalized along therapeutic lines but has the hidden agenda of retribution. Each person involved in the seclusion process should reflect upon their own motives and feelings with regard to seclusion use and the patient. 'Whistleblowing' (see Chapter 8) should begin at home.

ROLE OF CULTURE

The term culture is notoriously difficult to define and there are hundreds of published definitions. However, Leff (1988) manages to encompass the main concepts by saying, 'Culture encompasses all those aspects of human society that man has constructed or devised himself as opposed to those characteristics which are inborn'. It is, of course, difficult to define what is learned behaviour response and what is inherent. Yet culture can impinge on these inherent qualities and reshape them. It is perhaps not too surprising, in view of the coercive nature of psychiatry, that abuse of power occurs. Within the function of psychiatry there develops a subset of cultures based on ideologies, beliefs and values that are in the public domain.

The antipsychiatry lobby has been extremely articulate in

uncovering conceptual strands of the role psychiatry plays in society. Szasz (1962) set out an incisive argument regarding the dangers of a psychiatrized society, and stated: 'I submit that the traditional definition of psychiatry, which is still in vogue, places it alongside such things as alchemy and astrology, and commits it to the category of pseudo-science' (Szasz, 1962). Once psychiatry is institutionalized, either voluntarily or involuntarily, all the problems of total institutions (Goffman, 1968) lend themselves to the formation of specific cultures. Although Goffman was clear that institutional norms, rules and values did not wholly determine individual's actions, he did believe that they provided compelling material for the evolution of specific kinds of selves which form a 'group'. When patients are forced into psychiatric hospitals under legislative power, or coerced into them via social expectations (Parsons, 1951), they become extremely vulnerable to these institutional values.

Psychiatry, and hence psychiatric institutions, is seen to have a dual function: medical, and 'policing'. As Foucault (1988) puts it ' . . . and we psychiatrists are *the* functionaries of social order. It is up to us to make good these disorders. We have a function in public hygiene. That is the true vocation of psychiatry' (italics in the original). If this is true, then it is again not too surprising that, as agents of social order, hospital staff adopt mechanisms and strategies of control and dominance. It should be emphasized that these mechanisms take on a legitimacy, as they are derived from, and are rooted in, the wider society. Any culture has an invested interest in maintaining its position and existence, and attempts to dominate other cultures which impinge upon it. This 'cultural hegemony', a term coined by Antorio Gramsci, refers to the ' . . . precise ideas which are used at a particular time and place . . . to win the hearts and minds of the people over to an acceptance of the existing status quo' (Krause, 1977).

With the passage of time these institutional cultures form a tradition which adds greater force to the cultural values. The values, norms and beliefs become totemic (Levi-Strauss, 1962), symbolizing what each 'clan' represents, and routines and rituals develop that serve to display them. The seclusion of psychiatric patients can be viewed as an external sign of the ideologies of control and dominance that underlie the function of psychiatry.

As we saw earlier, in Eileen Morrison's (1990) study, the

'tradition of toughness' can develop as an institutional ethos within general psychiatric settings. Her article clearly identified the strutting machoism of nursing staff who perpetuated the image of control, who developed a representation of dominance and who openly portrayed pleasure when opportunities were provided in which control could be displayed. This form of cultural ideology is even more prominent in psychiatric institutions, where compulsorily detained patients are catered for in various degrees of security, for example within locked wards, regional and interim secure units and the special hospitals.

Richman and Mason (1992) report on nursing and culture from a British special hospital that caters for patients deemed to be dangerous, violent or having criminal propensities. One-third of the patient population are prison transfers. These authors argued that the cultural framework within the hospital was a 'mosaic' of prison mentality, failed treatment structures, a resultant time vacuum for the patients, and a conflict of treatment–security ideologies. Within this schemata nursing staff developed distancing techniques in order to prevent patients gaining knowledge of their personal lives, and patients became empowered when they gained such knowledge. They argued that 'Nursing groups maintain a tight frontier of control', and that ' . . . the special hospital nurse stands in a unique subculture and attempts to fulfil the medical promise, the nursing contract and the societal 'policing', in a type of order–conflict dimension' (Richman and Mason, 1992).

It is, of course, very difficult to care for patients who by their very nature can be violent and often dangerous. As was pointed out in Chapter 5, there may be a need for sanctions to control human populations; what should be asked, however, is whether seclusion should be one of those sanctions? If it is to be used, then we need to question whether there is a need to dismantle the cultural representation of seclusion as a controlling feature to maintain order. Seclusion abuse has occurred because those cultural values that have been affronted are punishable by the very people who have been hurt. Perhaps it is asking too much to expect people to constantly 'turn the other cheek' and not expect them to strike out in revenge. The seclusion of psychiatric patients may benefit from an independent assessment by those not emotionally and culturally involved, but also by those who appreciate the need to safeguard both patient and staff welfare.

CREATING VICTIMS

Given that abuse can and does occur, it must be understood that those who have been abused become victims of a practice which does more harm than good. New approaches to caring can often uncover and expose alarming situations which have difficult consequences, not just for the abused but also for those who are responsible for the abuse. After the discovery and acceptance that 'pindown' (Chapter 1) was an abusive intervention in childrens' homes, large amounts of compensation were paid by local authorities to the children involved, depending on how many days they were isolated as part of their 'treatment'.

Until recently, it was not thought that child sexual abuse had any effects on the children concerned. In a 1972 textbook entitled *Basic Psychiatry*, where psychology and psychiatric conditions are described simply for students, there is a brief outline about sexual assaults on children. The authors state: 'Contrary to expectations, even promiscuous children are relatively unaffected by their experiences . . . More commonly, the person who is most upset is the parent' (Sim and Gordon, 1972). Should this be said today there would be a public outcry, as deeper investigation into this problem has uncovered major psychological trauma within children who have been sexually abused. It may be that, as more insight is gained into seclusion, this practice will be viewed in the same light.

To finally label seclusion as an abuse, or to label some approaches to implementation of seclusion abusive, could cost the health authorities dear! Yet the psychological effects of abuse on the victims cannot be measured in monetary terms. No research has yet been carried out into the long-term effects of seclusion, yet if patients feel punished and violated these effects would be apparent. These may be post-traumatic stress syndrome or depression related to their sense of helplessness (Seligman, 1975). As anyone who has had their rights violated will know, this abuse may have far-reaching effects that may never be healed.

PREVENTING ABUSE

Recognizing that abuse occurs and taking steps to prevent it and monitor seclusion practice effectively are completely different matters. It is recognized by many that changes must take place, but to bring this about is difficult. Change may be effected by pressures from both within and without the organization or a combination of the two, but managers and carers have few options for altering care delivery.

The first response may be to ban seclusion altogether. The rationale behind this is obvious: if there is no seclusion practice there can be no seclusion abuse, and this is often argued as a viable alternative. Indeed, the Ashworth Inquiry findings stipulated that seclusion ought to be phased out of special hospital care completely. However, as we observed in Chapter 7, non-seclusion policies have their own problems. Lack of seclusion corresponds with higher medication rates and higher levels of stress among staff and patients.

A further response, preferred by most health authorities, is to use seclusion only as a last resort. Sadly, this too can fail, as this criterion is very difficult to quantify and vulnerable to individual interpretations, which can differ vastly during implementation. With this scenario more is said about when not to seclude patients than when seclusion is appropriate, and added to this is the fostering of 'false guilt' when seclusion is finally used, which adds to the general sense of negative emotions currently associated with seclusion use. Within this framework there are no standardized criteria for assessing when the use of seclusion is appropriate.

Another response is to relocate patients who would formerly have been placed in seclusion into other areas specially designed for the purpose. These may be police cells or specialist areas such as regional secure units (RSUs) which remove the patient from his immediate home area. It is even possible that known violent people are refused access to the ward because facilities are not available; they then return to the community, with the possible outcome of police involvement and maybe even criminal proceedings; this puts even further pressure on secure units and fails wholly to help the patient, who will be further segregated and stigmatized.

Gibson (1989) outlines three steps to prevent seclusion abuse, the first being to change nurses' attitudes towards seclusion. Gibson advocates experiential learning regarding the use of seclusion and their approach towards it, aimed at increasing nurses' sensitivity towards what seclusion entails. Antecedents to seclusion are to be particularly focused upon as a means of better understanding how seclusion is used. The second step in assisting prevention of abuse is to seek patients' views on seclusion and their perception of this. This should add to empathic understanding. Finally, Gibson points out that staffing levels ought to be kept adequate, and that should low staff levels be a reason for implementing seclusion this ought to be properly recorded on all incident sheets. These steps alone would indeed bring about some changes, but they do not provide a total picture of all the factors associated with change. Nonetheless, they would provide much material for assessment and reflection.

Hammill (1987) also attempts to describe practical ways to prevent seclusion abuse. These include four steps that can be adopted by any ward that practises seclusion, and will heighten awareness and understanding of the total picture necessary for sound decision making. Hammill recommends that patients ought to be given full explanations as to why seclusion was necessary, and should be made aware of the conditions under which seclusion would be terminated. She recommends that community meetings should focus on the issues surrounding seclusion and these be afforded an avenue for discussion between staff and patients. Finally, Hammill recommends that seclusion rooms ought to be 'as aesthetically pleasing as possible'. Again, the approaches adopted here are very limited, but once more discourse between nurses and between nurses and patients is highlighted as a valuable means of providing a better understanding.

MacDonald (1988) claims that organizational development is a necessary feature of management, and that outside influences can speed up the incrementalist change usually experienced within hospitals. As a manager responsible for a ward which appeared to use seclusion excessively (and may therefore be considered as abusing seclusion), he became concerned when the English National Board (ENB) refused to accept the ward as one of their training wards for student nurses. This resulted in an examination of the reasons why seclusion was practised too often. It was discovered that custodial concepts predominated among the staff implementing seclusion, and that little consensus was reached as to when seclusion should be implemented. Also, review procedures were very poor. MacDonald's approach involved many facets, but all with the express ideal of reducing seclusion hours. The first action involved changing the name of the ward from 'secure purposes' to 'intensive care', and this was quickly followed by reviewing the seclusion procedure itself. This resulted in all seclusions requiring a precise clinical reason, regular reviews and checks by both nursing and medical staff, plus a full team review once seclusion was terminated. Staff numbers were also increased and the skills mix was changed. Other measures included changing the ward decor and furnishings. Although this approach to reducing seclusion hours was forced upon the organization and implemented by non-ward based managers, it once again transpired that debriefing sessions were extremely useful in 'skills and attitudinal development' (MacDonald, 1988), which proved to be the most vital prerequisite for change to take place. Eventually, the incidence of seclusion in this area was reduced from 130 per month to fewer than five. While outside influence in effecting change is welcomed, it would still appear to be more advantageous for the caring professions to assess care strategies at ward level. The ENB did eventually accept the above ward on the training circuit, but it is sad that such a severe measure was not anticipated by the managers concerned. It is quite possible that morale had failed long before the sanction was implemented, and that this had never been noticed by the managers concerned. It behoves managers to anticipate and support change before outside influences intervene.

CHANGING SECLUSION PRACTICE

The whole ethos of health care delivery has changed and is continuing to change, with nurses and health care workers being expected to adjust to and even anticipate changes in response to social, political, technological and economic trends. The whole context of seclusion practice reflects the pressure from these trends.

Central government attempts to address these issues by implementing policies aimed at improving and raising standards of health care. In theory, these new approaches are expected to protect and safeguard patients and patients become the focus of caring; in practice, health care workers are left with a balancing act between the top-down approach of management strategies for implementing change and hearing and meeting the demands of the patients in their care. Because a nurse has 'hands-on' care in a unique and intimate relationship with her patients, she alone has specialist knowledge, which must temper and facilitate any changes intended to meet the needs of both the people she works for and the people she cares for. Changing seclusion practice is difficult within this kind of setting.

Clay (1986) points out that 'The structure of the profession and the role of the nurse as a health care professional has almost all been determined with the assistance of external agencies'. In other words, legal, societal and medical developments impinge on nursing practice and force change upon nurses. Nurses find it very difficult to effect change alone without the help of these external agencies, even when they have little or no concept of the difficulties facing practitioners when implementing new policies.

Owen (1988) points out that 'Change implies the break up of existing patterns and the formulation of new ones and is not complete until these are established'. Wright (1989) goes on to define this further by describing change as 'An attempt to alter or replace existing knowledge, skills, attitudes, norms and styles of individuals and groups. It is a discontinuity of the subjects' past behaviours and their perception of that discontinuity'. The effect of change within mental health and seclusion has, however, been piecemeal, and the fact that this is the first book to address this emotive subject reflects this. Some units have made great leaps forward in attempting to address the issue, with some even banning seclusion completely, but this is not occurring at all levels of practice and in all situations. On the whole, seclusion practice is undergoing a change, and is only at the beginning of the process. Everyone knows that something ought to be done, but no-one seems to know what it should be. The fact that most inquiries into seclusion practice fail to incorporate known ethical components in analysis highlights the fact that this dismantling of existing patterns has never completely taken place.

RESISTANCE TO CHANGE

There has been much resistance to change in practice. Kotter and Schlesinger (cited in Thomas, 1988) explain four reasons for this resistance. The first is a desire not to lose something, such as influence, money or status. In the case of seclusion, there are great difficulties where a custodial approach to care has been adopted. To keep someone in custody implies that the custodians have access to some power or influence which the patient does not. This authoritarian approach to care cannot simply be altered by individuals being told to accept patients as equals. The second reason is misunderstanding or lack of trust in those bringing in the change: for some reason (surprising in a profession which deals with people) nurse managers can be remarkably poor communicators; there is often suspicion underlying communications between nurses and their managers, and a tendency for nurses to pay only lip-service to proposed changes, which are then weak and ineffective. The third reason for resistance is a belief that the change does not make sense for the organization, i.e. others do not share the same understanding of the situation as those introducing the change, or do not have the same priorities in mind. A manager may be calling for seclusion hours to be reduced and the nursing staff feel threatened and tense on the wards because they feel a safe way of dealing with aggression is now unavailable to them. It is not surprising that resistance will occur and morale may suffer. Finally, there is currently a low tolerance of change in health care services, due to rapid successive changes which have led to low morale. Changes in education, funding and management, as well as changes in technology and practice, have all added to the stress of an already stressful work environment. This has led to unease among care providers, who feel that the stability of old practices and approaches has gone.

Wright (1989) argues that there are further reasons for resistance within nursing, these being 'Fear of the unknown, competition for power or influence, and limited resources'. These are wholly applicable to seclusion practice. First, fear of the unknown will cause a great amount of consternation. Nurses who are inadequately prepared in using alternative strategies for dealing with violence and hyperstimulation will no doubt experience some disquiet at facing such a situation without recourse to seclusion. Past experience has taught them that this is the only safe way of dealing with a disruptive and disturbed individual, and there is understandable fear of the unknown outcomes of assessing situations differently. Secondly, competition for power or influence will make changing seclusion practice very difficult. If practitioners are told that someone else has decided that seclusion is wrong and ought not to be implemented, or that it must not be implemented in particular situations, then natural resistance will occur. Not only will the power associated with the implementation be denied, but the fact that others are dictating their own practice will make them feel particularly uncomfortable, and be seen as an infringement of the nursing role.

The final category of limited resources leading to resistance is applicable in that further training and possibly higher staff ratios will be deemed necessary if seclusion abuse is to be prevented. Ward managers, who are now deemed to be budget-holders, may resist such investment should other, more pressing, factors vie for funding. Indeed, these influences have the potential to greatly impede any change in seclusion practice and must be given due consideration.

Clay (1986) feels that this resistance to change has begun at far deeper levels than described above. He feels that such resistance is indicative of the philosophical approaches to care which have been valued by nurses over the past century. Unfortunately, these philosophies have all created barriers to change which must be understood and addressed. Clay describes four philosophical approaches and explores them in relation to change within nursing, the first being romanticism, which values hierarchical structures and idealizes the nurse as handmaid to doctors. The second, pragmatism, also hinders change in that the nurse is held to be there to help the doctor in task allocation. The emphasis is on training rather than an understanding or knowledge of practice. It is pragmatism that led to patients being seen as 'conditions', which is so decried in nursing literature today. The third philosophical approach, humanism, presents its own problems and challenges. Humanism began to reject the medical, pragmatic approach, but in Britain nursing still appears to be beholden to the medical model for its approach. Humanism has led to the call for autonomy within nursing and nurses as practitioners who can take into account the whole person. The final philosophy is existentialism. This upholds the rights of the patient to refuse or accept treatment, and focuses on the responsibility of the nurse to be accountable first to the patient in her care. This has developed over the past 10–15 years, and has led to such approaches as primary nursing and the named nurse.

As these philosophies have developed, so have the difficulties in bringing about changes in mental health care, because there are often no direct cause and effect approaches to mental health difficulties. The philosophies outlined by Clay are very important in addressing the issues surrounding seclusion practice, and all are apparent within psychiatric practice.

Since the 1940s, when mental health nursing was combined with general nurse training, there has been over-emphasis and reliance on the medical profession to lead the way in treatment modalities. The psychiatric nurse contained the situation on the wards in between times, and any visitor to these old 'asylums' will appreciate that containment was all that could be expected, as single nurses were often left in charge of hundreds of patients on locked units. One of the authors talked to a nursing sister who had worked in such a hospital in the 1930s. She described building fires as being the main priority on winter mornings, having to carry huge buckets of coal up four flights of stairs. This sister described having certain 'trustees' (patients who helped with the general running of the ward) who, in her opinion, were no longer ill but could no longer live outside the hospital. Simple human interactions always took place in the company of a hundred other people, and basic hygiene was never private. Bathtime was particularly traumatic for this nurse: patients had to strip in a locked corridor then, opening the door, the trustees allowed a few patients through at a time. Each patient was unceremoniously bathed (without changing the water) and then sent into another locked corridor area to be dried and dressed. With 200 patients to bathe weekly this was all that could be done. Violence was common and a good trustee was a valuable asset when medication was so limited. Added to basic patient care was responsibility for cleaning, which was regularly checked by senior staff.

All in all, mental health nursing has undergone a transformation since that time, yet this dependence on medical staff for diagnosis etc. continues. In areas where seclusion is carried out it is doctors who bear the responsibility for deciding whether seclusion is to continue. Pragmatism also added to this philosophical approach, and patients continued to be depersonalized, known only by their previous history and behaviour. However, humanism has brought about major shifts in thinking about seclusion practice, with many articles being written in this philosophical style (Barradell, 1985). As humanism evolved it became more understandable that patients, no matter how ill, could make their own decisions about life. Unfortunately, when someone is becoming violent it is unacceptable to sit by and allow their aggression to damage themselves or others, and this conflicts strongly with the more modern philosophies of nursing. As Clay points out, change is less able to occur when all these philosophies coexist and conflict. Nowhere is this more obvious than in seclusion practice.

Change is necessary when one considers the hotchpotch of approaches implemented when applying seclusion practice, but there should be a clear understanding of what is to be changed and why. So far, there is little agreement among practitioners as to what is necessary for change to occur and, more importantly, for change to become established and effective, with real progress being the outcome in the long term. Change is a 'buzzword' of the 1990s and becomes an accepted part of nursing management strategy, yet we must take care that change actually occurs, and is not simply discussed, planned and never realized.

10

Ethical issues

Ann Alty

If literature on seclusion is lacking then literature dealing with the ethical issues or principles underpinning the implementation of seclusion is even more scarce. However, ethical debate surrounding nursing practice is imperative. It has been pointed out that 'Ethical reasoning can present the nurse with a means of enhancing the decision making process involved in the delivery of care' (Kendrick, 1991).

Ethical studies regarding seclusion to date are extremely few: opinions and anecdotal evidence seem to make up the bulk of the literature base. Gibson (1989) rightly points out that 'Much of psychiatry is as yet unexplained – consequently, psychiatric practices have always provoked some controversy'. Seclusion does seem to be one of these areas, provoking emotive reactions on both sides. It is interesting to observe that many who argue for the use of seclusion use theoretical bases for their points, whereas those who argue against seclusion use moral or anecdotal evidence.

Much of the literature regarding ethical issues of seclusion is invalid as considered studies point the way forward towards better research-based practice. It appears to be emotive and unconsidered as ethical reasoning. Indeed, one article often cited by others as a valuable ethical contribution to the seclusion debate makes a completely emotive argument which has little to do with quality of care or practice. The writer uses statements such as 'Their caretakers plunge them into a darker night than they ever knew' (Pilette, 1978). While this is a graphic attempt to draw attention to the plight of the patient in seclusion, it serves to divide opinion rather than to examine it helpfully, and says little to dissuade others from using seclusion other than perhaps to create a false sense of guilt!

It could be argued that the use of policies and guidelines has also contributed to this vagueness. Such guidelines are usually set up by bodies or health authorities for those who practise seclusion (RCN, 1979; Ritter, 1989), and usually lack ethical or moral implications, generally focusing on the legal rights of both nurse and patient as well as safety in implementation. Indeed, most seem to deliberately avoid the moral debate while acknowledging that it exists, and choose instead to hold neutral ground. However, in the absence of alternative treatment or practice they uphold the use of seclusion by providing officially approved guidelines. It could be argued that providing such guidelines allows nurses to continue to implement seclusion without questioning their motives or reasons. Their trust in the advisory body permits seclusion to become accepted practice, as neither party takes responsibility for examining the evidence. A false sense of security in the value of the practice therefore arises – the managers provide guidelines because nurses use seclusion, and nurses use seclusion because the managers provide guidelines. As has been pointed out: 'A preoccupation with legal requirements and with procedural guidelines, and an appeal to such as the ultimate arbiters of morality, is seen as detrimental to the more humane, soul searching inquiry prompted by ethical reflection' (McGovern, 1991).

[Ethical reflection is never comfortable. Nor is it a simple 'black or white' reasoning process. However, it is a necessary basis for reflection which shifts or enlightens values and attitudes towards behaviour or practice. In the case of seclusion, nurses are the people working closest to the patient in order to bring therapeutic input. Nurses must therefore take responsibility for examining the facts surrounding seclusion for themselves. This will involve ethical reflection in order to better understand the practice and recommend future care. Hopefully, this will bring about changes in attitudes towards seclusion as well as providing a better established basis for practice which could provide the answers to more searching questions. As has already been pointed out, the fact that the procedure exists may not be valid as a reason to continue, and nurses need now, more than ever, to examine seclusion in a way which reflects nursing development at this time. As described previously, it is nurses who are best in a position to voice these issues: 'Change, if it is to occur, must first occur with nurses' (Craig, Ray and Hix, 1989). Facilitating such change is never simple, yet it is important to view the practice of seclusion as having potential to benefit by change concerning ethical reasoning.⌉

It is extremely difficult to actually define what ethical reasoning is in relation to practice, and more often than not this kind of debate is left to those who are felt to be 'out of touch' with clinical practice. Any subsequent ethical debate is therefore often discounted as being inapplicable to the practice situation: practitioners adopt the approach that those engaging in named ethical research are unable to apply it to ward practice. Seclusion is one of these areas. While much is made of legal rights and safe guidelines, little is made of the ethical or philosophical issues which surround seclusion. This is probably because nursing has been greatly influenced by the scientific approach of the medical model, with its emphasis upon causal relationships, task allocation and routinization (Pearson and Vaughan, 1986). The medical model of care is strongly criticized by Szasz (1973), as is the fact that the medical approach denies any recourse to philosophical contemplation and reflection. He states: 'Because psychiatrists avoid taking a forthright and responsible stand on the problems they deal with, the major intellectual and moral predicaments of psychiatry remain unacknowledged and unexamined'. Indeed, Szasz' argument points out that ethical and moral examination is never part of the psychiatrist's care of the patient, and while this is possibly an extreme conclusion to reach it does bear some truth, as more recent writers have stated that ethical codes of conduct within psychiatry may be self-protecting rather than liberating (Barker and Baldwin, 1991). Ethical discourse within psychiatry is therefore difficult due to the hazy boundaries, and possibly the unwillingness of some practitioners to examine their own motives and thoughts.

Ethics cannot create hard and fast rules for practice but they are extremely important, as everyone engages in ethical reasoning at some time and all nurses encounter situations which involve moral thought or action. Others take this argument even further and claim that 'All our actions pose an ethical question' (Barker and Baldwin, 1991), as has been pointed out: 'The word ethics is notoriously ambiguous and a precise definition cannot be given. However, one of its meanings is 'The philosophical study of moral conduct and reasoning' ' (Sparkes, 1991).

Philosophical study is extremely useful for a better understanding of the debate surrounding seclusion. Philosophy is not something which can be rendered available and understandable only by the deep thinker, who composes hypotheses using metaphysical statements and concepts which bear no relation to everyday nursing, but may be regarded as 'essentially the act of clarification' (Seedhouse, 1986). Therefore it is not an end in itself, but merely a tool to facilitate clearer thinking: one considers the practice situation, then reflects philosophically before applying any reflection to practice. The study of seclusion can be greatly assisted by philosophical and ethical reasoning. Philosophy is largely involved in asking questions which may, at first, seem obvious. However, on closer scrutiny this questioning may illuminate practice in a way which could strengthen the reasoning behind it, and protect the perhaps necessary use of seclusion in British psychiatric hospitals and units. Such reflection may subsequently lead to care which better protects patients.

Questions regarding seclusion are seldom asked aloud, and rarely are they open to discussion or consideration in the structure of everyday psychiatric practice. These questions may indeed be relatively simplistic and could thus be overlooked, because they appear at first to stem from ignorance. They may include: 'Why is seclusion carried out?' 'Is seclusion helpful?' 'Is it wrong to force someone into a room with no means of escape when they have done nothing wrong other than to be ill?' These and other questions will have within them some ethical concepts which have already been addressed at length in ethical and philosophical works. Some of these concepts include autonomy, respect, paternalism, rights, beneficence and non-maleficence. It is hoped that a brief examination of these concepts with regard to seclusion will provoke thought and further discussion, which will clarify current thought and practice and, if necessary, expose discrepancies and problems within the practice of seclusion itself.

AUTONOMY AND SECLUSION

Autonomy is a crucial area for discussion in relation to seclusion, and is closely linked with assessment of competency and respect for persons (Downie and Calman, 1987). When someone is said to be acting or behaving autonomously it refers to his 'ability to be self-governing' (Kendrick, 1991). It is seen as incorporating two distinct areas, 'self-determination' and 'self-government' (Atkinson, 1991). Self-determination is a key issue within the debate as it 'involves individuals being able to formulate and carry out their own plans, desires, wishes and policies, thereby determining the course of their own life' (Atkinson, 1991). In many respects it could be argued that this is ignored or overridden when a mentally ill adult is locked within a seclusion room. Indeed, it is difficult to see how the patient in seclusion is being allowed to formulate and carry out his own plans, desires, wishes and policies, as at this point in time control is definitely placed in the hands of the nurse who holds the keys and the doctors who may enforce medication to control the situation.

The fact that the patient is placed in seclusion implies that he is, to some degree, considered to be incompetent and incapable of self-government. Much enforced intervention within psychiatry is either explicitly or implicitly linked with judgements by staff as to whether the individual is competent to formulate plans related to self-determination and self-government. Roth, Meisel and Lidz (1983) outline five understood 'tests' for competency, which are: evidencing a choice and preference for or against treatment; reasonable outcome of choice (i.e. evaluating the patient's capacity to reach responsible or right choices); choice based on 'rational reasons' (i.e. whether the choice is a result of mental illness); ability to understand the outcomes of the choice; and actual understanding of the choice. Within these tests unwise choices are permitted providing they do not encroach on others' autonomy. It is understood in psychiatry that when the patient is disruptive or aggressive and clearly evidencing hallucinations that impair rational decision-making or understanding of the situation, staff may use seclusion as a means of containment until a measure of competency returns. Of course, 'rational' reasons and 'reasonable' outcome of choice imply that competency is measured against norms which may differ between persons and cultures, and calls are made to assess patients carefully in relation to their culture (Jorsh, 1991). Indeed, it has been pointed out that seclusion is used more readily for black people (Fernando, 1991). Judgements made by staff concerning an individual's competency are therefore often subjective, without standardization and extremely difficult to measure effectively.

The concept of respecting the individual's autonomy and ability to make choices leads the discussion to the area of 'respect for persons'.

Respect for persons may be regarded as a continuum with no respect at one end and full respect at the other. An individual may be treated to some measure of respect at any time, but this may not be the full respect that is given to the mature, self-governing individual. Full respect, and therefore full autonomy, is only given to those who are judged to be behaving competently and maturely. The way a patient is perceived by staff may have a bearing on the decision to seclude. He may be described as being not fully a person when he behaves abnormally. Person-hood is a much-debated philosophical issue, and lack of person-hood may be intimated by the patient's carers; for example, when a violent patient is described as 'not being himself' or judged by statements such as 'He acted like an animal', this may reflect a decision to no longer consider the individual as a person and therefore legitimize any abuse of the respect that would normally be afforded him or her. It is within this context that the violently psychotic individual is denied full respect and autonomy, although some respect will still be afforded relative to his actions and his situation.

Confusion often arises within this context when the words 'dignity' and 'respect' are used interchangeably. The two are, in fact, discrete, and it is worth noting that it is possible to uphold dignity while denying full respect for the person. A patient can be treated in a dignified way within seclusion even though he is judged to be incompetent. Often, abuse of the patient lies not in the fact that he was secluded but in *how* the process was carried out. To seclude someone may be necessary and can be dealt with in a professional and dignified manner. Preservation of dignity is one way of ensuring that the patient is not devalued as an individual during the seclusion process.

Singer (1979) cites Fletcher's indictors of personhood for discussion, these being self-awareness, a sense of future, a sense of past, the capacity to relate to others, concern for others, communication and curiosity. It is argued that someone must have all these indicators intact to be perceived as a person. When a patient is behaving violently towards either himself or others, it could be argued that he is not behaving in the fullest sense of humanhood as many of these indicators are not apparent. Others, however, prefer more simplistic definitions. One of the basic characteristics of personhood is to 'have the ability of future development' (Seedhouse, 1988). This indicates that personhood is a 'process' rather than having measurable indicators, and it could be argued that the person who is acutely violent due to mental illness is actually no less a person because he may indeed have the ability to develop understanding and awareness after the episode or perhaps even because of the episode. On this premise it may be argued that the individual is entitled to complete respect and full autonomy in whatever state he is. On the other hand, it could be argued (and is often felt) that at the moment of the incident, particularly where the individual is psychotic, the patient has ceased to develop as a person for that given time. Seclusion will thus be used to contain the situation while the individual endeavours to recommence development. This would coincide with the argument discussed earlier on the use of seclusion as a way of providing ego restraints until the patient can do so for himself. In this case, the ego could be seen to be the particular area necessary for development as a person, and that domination by basic instinct (id) or superego constraints is not appropriate to valuable development as a person.

Of course, it is argued that we never have complete autonomy, as there are societal constraints and responsibilities which might override the individual's wishes, plans and desires (Atkinson, 1991). In the case of seclusion these restrictions are obvious, and in addition other people (i.e. nurses, psychologists and medical staff) make decisions as to whether the individual patient remains within seclusion or is returned to the ward area. The patient is thus stripped of his autonomy and his ability to govern himself. Interestingly, it could be argued that the patient is still able to govern his ability from within his locked environment, even though it is extremely limited. He can choose to be violent or regain his composure, and this may be facilitated by medication. Once he regains this composure, the fact that he can behave autonomously within this locked environment ensures that the decision will be taken to release the patient.

An interesting consideration in relation to this is the fact that autonomy may be overridden in the short term to ensure long-term autonomy for the patient (Atkinson, 1991): for example, a suicidal patient may be restrained within seclusion, thereby having his short-term autonomy curtailed to give him back his long-term autonomy when the suicidal episode is passed. A further example might be a seriously violent or homicidal patient who is briefly stripped of his autonomy in order to prevent him having his long-term autonomy curtailed by being placed on a murder charge, should he actually be allowed to murder someone else. It might be worth regarding seclusion in terms of this 'short-term' or 'long-term' autonomy, as the short term may have significant bearing on the long term. Those who argue for defence of liberty are usually basing their argument on the fact that autonomy is the most valued aspect of man. However, immediate autonomy may not be the dominant ethic when other factors are considered.

The problem is that mental illness often affects personality or cognition, or both, and in this case the patient may be judged to be behaving in a non-autonomous fashion, particularly when the change is drastic. Full autonomy only exists where there is full knowledge of the facts. Indeed, it has been argued that 'all illness represents a state of diminished autonomy' (Komrad, 1983) and, as has been described above, it is often difficult to determine whether any person ever does have full knowledge of his own circumstances in order to reach decisions about his self-determination.

PATERNALISM AND SECLUSION

Some argue that paternalism is wrong as an attitude within health care; however, in situations where it is debatable whether or not a person has full knowledge of his own situation, or where autonomy is perceived to be restricted, paternalism will arise, usually where there is little time or where a 'fixed false belief' is held (Atkinson, 1991). It is clearly understood in the case of seclusion that the situation is often an emergency, and also often involves people whose beliefs are fixed and false (as with delusions, hallucinations or paranoia). With this definition seclusion ought to be underlined as an area where paternalism will be raised again and again.

When a patient is behaving violently or threatening violence there is very little time for staff to make a decision as to the care necessary at this time. It has been indicated by research that supervision of such patients is very stressful (Jones *et al.*, 1987).

In such a highly charged atmosphere it is probable that people will react quickly, and the first issue will be that of safety – safety of the violent patient, safety of the general ward population and safety of members of staff. In this situation paternalism may become the attitude that dominates the decision. The patient will be placed in seclusion 'for his own good' or 'for the good of others around him', and his full autonomy will be affected by paternalism.

Unfortunately, this may be abused by the staff in the form of 'unrestrained paternalism' (Atkinson, 1991), where the patient's autonomy is eroded unnecessarily to the point of causing harm to his wellbeing. Interestingly, Wulff, Pederson and Rosenberg (1991) divide paternalism into three categories, and these are very useful when discussing paternalism in relation to seclusion.

The first category, that of 'genuine paternalism' is wholly supported in Wulff's argument. He feels that, in certain cases (i.e. where the patient is unconscious, delirious or severely mentally handicapped), it is perfectly understandable to take decisions for the patient because autonomy is already greatly diminished. The second category, that of 'solicited paternalism' lies in the relationship between care providers and patients. The patient and nurse understand that in some areas the nurse will decide the course of action, and the patient is willing to go along with this. This, he argues, is as morally acceptable as the first category and is related to explicit or implicit consent to an act by the patient. The third category: that of 'unsolicited paternalism', is the area where Wulff feels there are serious ethical problems, where neither of the above two categories applies. He goes on to point out:

> 'The difficulty consists in drawing the line between unsolicited and solicited paternalism, and there is a great need for public debate and descriptive ethical studies which may show what people expect, when, for instance, they are admitted to hospital. This is the only way to establish those generally accepted norms which are needed to guide medical practitioners.' (Wulff, Pederson and Rosenberg, 1990).

Paternalism in relation to seclusion may fit into any of those categories. For example, genuine paternalism may arise with the seriously psychotic patient who is out of control and determined to carry out what his hallucinations indicate. It may also arise on the acute psychiatric unit, where someone is admitted and suspected of being under the influence of mind-altering illicit drugs and behaving violently. This type of paternalism is morally justified when considering the options available to the nurse in caring for someone in such a severely distressed state. Whether this paternalism is demonstrated by locking the patient in seclusion, however, is debatable and must be considered against other criteria.

The second category, that of 'solicited paternalism' often occurs in hospital, where a patient may ask to enter seclusion. There are also studies which demonstrate that, while patients originally objected to being placed in seclusion, they fully supported that action when they were finally well. In these cases nurses may be acting on implicit consent, which is later understood by all concerned to have been helpful at the time.

The final category, unsolicited paternalism, may also apply to care within a psychiatric unit or hospital. Here the nurse may act intuitively, thinking she has made the right decision to seclude. However, this decision may be wrong and never identified as such, while considerable pain and moral injury has been inflicted on the patient. The nurse may have mistakenly felt that the patient had implicitly given consent, and acted on that feeling. Alternatively, the patient who constantly asks for seclusion is not always choosing the best option for himself. Placing such a patient into seclusion may underline his lack of autonomy and further reinforce paternalism, which is wrongly applied in the given situation. The difficulty lies in whether or not it is possible to draw the line between the two categories. It takes an experienced nurse to do so, and she must balance her knowledge of the patient with her awareness of the situation and her intuitive moral understanding. Much is therefore open to error or misjudgment on the nurse's part. Misunderstandings and misinterpretations may lead to serious moral trauma for the patient.

It has been pointed out that when superiority, domination, oppression and dogmatism are present this actually amounts to 'authoritarianism' and has no relationship to true paternalism, which is always helpful to the patient (Komrad, 1983). Unsolicited paternalism may therefore be classified as authoritarianism, and this will sometimes happen when the adult mentally ill person is placed in seclusion. This is an area of much debate for those who are completely against seclusion. It is argued that the abuse of the situation must be prevented by preventing *all* seclusion. A total ban on seclusion would prevent any misuse or abuse, but it would also limit the options available to the nurse, who would use the practice widely in a way that is completely morally substantiated.

BENEFICENCE, NON-MALEFICENCE AND SECLUSION

The principles of beneficence and non-maleficence raise much debate in the discussion surrounding seclusion. It is important to ascertain whether the procedure of seclusion is helpful or not to the patient. Much of this debate is centred on these two areas, and becomes polarized into two camps. Some claim that seclusion is never morally justified (Pilette, 1978; Sallah, 1992), while others state that seclusion is helpful and even good for the patient in certain circumstances (Miller, 1992). Indeed, non-maleficence and beneficence are cited by Downie and Calman (1987) in four principles of what they call 'consensus morality'. The first definition is that 'One ought not to harm other people physically or psychologically' (non-maleficence) and that 'One ought to give positive help to people wherever necessary' (beneficence). O'Brien (1989) points out that 'Placing a patient in seclusion is often painful, frightening and apprehensive for both clients and staff', and Myers (1990) agrees that there are harmful effects of seclusion which include the possibility of setting up an 'aggression cycle' which can escalate within the ward (Van Ryb-roek *et al.*, 1987). Indeed, it has been said that seclusion is a means for the staff to act out their own feelings of helplessness and fear when faced with a violent individual (Hodgkinson, 1985), which has nothing to do with either beneficence or non-maleficence. If these observations are true, then beneficence and non-maleficence as described above have been violated.

At the end of 1991 a nursing journal published an article on seclusion which basically asked what all the fuss was about (Brennan, 1991). A series of letters and articles arguing about these principles followed. One writer states: 'Nurses should be aware that the worst injustices perpetrated by one person against another can be hidden behind the facade of therapeutic care', and goes on to state that 'The nurse has a duty to do what is best for each individual patient' (Sallah, 1992). In effect, Sallah was arguing about the two issues of non-maleficence and beneficence. He felt that seclusion was unhelpful and even damaging to the patient's wellbeing in the long term. In research it has even been linked to punishment (Whaley and Ramirez, 1980). Alternatively, Brennan (1991) feels that seclusion can be a positive, helpful intervention and this is upheld by Campbell, Shepard and Falconer (1982) and Gutheil (1978), who feel that using seclusion is as helpful as a means of reducing stimulation for the already disturbed patient and achieving safety for other patients and staff.

Studies of patient responses provide equally conflicting evidence. When asked if a seclusion room was necessary on the ward, 76% of secluded patients and 93% of non-secluded patients said 'Yes' (Hammill, 1987). However, when individuals were asked about their own seclusion experience the response was divided, with 60% of those who observed seclusion being used expressing negative feelings towards staff. Helplessness, disgust, depression and anger have also been reported (Heyman, 1987). In a further study patients felt they had experienced angry and sad feelings while in seclusion, and scored lowest on those ratings that indicated the patient felt protected and safe (Hammill *et al.*, 1989). Another study demonstrated that nurses and patients significantly disagreed about the feelings of secluded patients, and that nurses should never make assumptions about patients' attitudes (Richardson, 1987). (For a further analysis of these studies see Chapter 11.) Some have reported successful non-seclusion policies, as they feel that 'a seriously disturbed patient should not be left alone' (Kingdon and Bakewell, 1988).

With the above discrepancies in mind it is difficult to ascertain whether seclusion is helpful or not, and it has been underlined that little valid evidence actually testifies to its effectiveness as a form of containment and reduction of stimulation (Hodgkinson, 1985; Angold, 1989). Also, confusion over outcomes occurs because often seclusion and medication are used concurrently making it impossible to pinpoint which of the two interventions is being measured.

RIGHTS AND SECLUSION

Linking all the ethical principles surrounding seclusion is the issue of rights. It has been pointed out that 'rights and duties can be seen as the opposite sides of the same coin' (Burnard and Chapman, 1988), which leads to the conclusion that, within nursing, if a patient has a right then the nurse has a duty to uphold that right. However, nurses also have rights, which can also be violated by those around them, including patients.

The notion of 'rights' may have different emphases in different disciplines, for example, legal rights may differ from moral rights. Beauchamp and Childress (1983) point out that 'legal rights are claims that are justified by legal principles and rules, and moral rights are claims that are justified by moral principles and rules' (Beauchamp and Childress, 1983). Nonetheless, it is difficult to discuss rights without saying what right the person in question has and outlining who it is that has the duty to provide and uphold those rights (Raz, 1986).

A simple explanation of the term rights is that moral theories may be expressed in terms of rights, and it has been pointed out that talking about rights is simply an alternative way to express what is meant in terms of principles. In consequence, rights are the results of rules or principles, and the moral rights discussed in ethics are merely 'One way of expressing moral principles' (Downie and Calman, 1987). Therefore, a patient has a right to be treated in a dignified way, expressing the principle of value for individuals, and the nurse has a duty to uphold and protect this right of her patient. Within seclusion practice it is extremely difficult to determine exactly which rights and principles are to be upheld, because it has never actually been established what rights a patient does have within seclusion.

It has been pointed out that 'The rights of the mentally ill are problematic because the humanity of those who have lost the capacity to reason may be questioned' (Campbell, 1986). Legal rights do not necessarily uphold moral rights, but serve to underpin and protect those moral rights which have been identified as being worthy of upholding. There remains some difficulty in affording the mentally ill the status of personhood and the full autonomy which goes with that, and there have been no established legal rights afforded the patient within seclusion since the Lunacy Act of 1890. Campbell goes on to point out that 'even the most general rhetoric of human rights, although explicitly universalistic, seems to harbour the basis for depriving the mentally ill of fundamental rights' (Campbell, 1986). It could be argued that in the case of the mentally ill there is much confusion as to their status, and therefore their valid rights and the upholding of these. Many declarations of human rights use ambiguous phrases concerning the mentally ill, and this has contributed little to the debate and accentuated the confusion. For example, Article 5 of the United Nations Universal Declaration of Human Rights states: 'No-one shall be subjected to torture or to cruel, inhuman or degrading treatment or punishment' (HMSO, 1984), but the subsequent exploration in relation to British human rights completely fails to address mental illness.

The recent Patient's Charter has been strongly criticized by Robin Cook, the then Labour health spokesman, who said: 'No charter will work if patients have no real means of demanding their rights' (Millar, 1991). Although stating that patients have certain rights, there is no structured means for the patient to pursue those rights, nor for those who care for him to act as advocates. Codes of conduct continually stress the right of the patient to autonomy but, as has been pointed out, there is a considerable discrepancy between philosophical outlines of care and the actual care given (Beardshaw, 1981).

Linked into the issue of rights is the often neglected area of nurses' rights. When a patient is behaving violently nurses should have the right to protect themselves. Mill (1962) argued that self-protection warranted interference and control, in order to prevent harm to others. Possibly more than one in ten psychiatric patients assault staff (Schipperheijn and Dunne, 1991) and many of these assaults go unreported for various reasons. It has been pointed out that 'working in a psychiatric hospital amounts to consent to be assaulted' (Stilling, 1992), but this is surely a problem which has not been sufficiently addressed in relation to seclusion. It is possible that by not using seclusion the nurses put themselves at considerable risk of physical harm and emotional stress. Many nurses feel that this goes with the job, but Stilling argues that this is not necessarily the correct way to think. As has been pointed out, 'All people have a primary need for experiencing protection from bodily harm' (Beauchamp and Childress, 1983), yet nurses are often denied the right to fulfil this basic need, because they are expected to be benign and unassertive. Where disturbed or agitated behaviour occurs on the ward setting it will constantly cause a conflict in rights which nurses must address. To do this accurately and expertly, nurses must have considerable understanding of any given situation they may be in. If threatened by violence outside the hospital, nurses will be as vulnerable as the next person with a right to protect themselves, yet within the hospital setting nurses must shift their moral code to deny themselves a basic human instinct for self-preservation.

SUMMARY

Ethical discourse concerning the seclusion of mentally ill patients is imperative if steps are to be taken to improve care. Those arguments already contributed to the debate are couched in emotional terms which do much to confuse the issue rather than clarify it. Ethical and philosophical debate, carried out responsibly, ought to make the known facts clearer and help towards decision-making. It is vital to future seclusion care that the ethical points raised briefly here, be applied more rigorously to the debate. The fact that people have not yet developed better ethical discourse surrounding seclusion practice has helped to keep the practice hidden, and therefore fraught with dangers. It is hoped that future research will pay much more regard to ethical and philosophical principles in exploring this issue.

11

Patients' views about seclusion

Ann Alty and Tom Mason

So far in this book the authors have focused on the academic study of seclusion practice and the professional issues pertaining to its use. However, it is our opinion that any study of seclusion is void unless patients' perception and experience are taken into account. For many reasons, some which have been discussed in previous chapters, the views of patients are very often ignored, minimized or marginalized by professionals in the field of mental health. Indeed, in a literature search carried out by the authors, only 12 articles were discovered which seriously addressed the issue of patients' feelings within seclusion. Shields (1985) argues that this failure to appreciate patients' views is 'a prominent feature of the reduced social status of being a psychiatric patient', and this is highly likely to be the main reason why patients' views are not sought. Goffman (1963) described stigmas as being attributes which discredit and devalue the individual, and Teasdale (1987) points out that the stigma of being labelled 'mentally ill' is 'deeply ingrained' in western society. Also it has been noted that nurses are resistant to patient feedback (Shields, Morrison and Hart, 1988) and perceive patient involvement as criticism, finding this threatening both professionally and personally.

NURSES' PERCEPTIONS AND SECLUSION

Throughout the available research papers it is underlined that nurses often do not perceive how a patient feels when placed in seclusion. There is often a disparity in perception between nurses and patients, with patients indicating more painful experiences than those described by nurses (Hammill *et al.*, 1989; Binder and McCoy, 1983; Soliday, 1985). There is evidence to show that staff see seclusion as punishment for behaviours which are considered to be unacceptable (Whaley and Ramirez, 1980).

FEELINGS WITHIN SECLUSION

Binder and McCoy (1983) found that the majority of patients in their study felt there was absolutely nothing good about their experiences of seclusion. A literature search of 12 available articles uncovered a total of 33 identified feelings of patients while placed in seclusion (see Table 11.1). Of these, only 18 were identified more than once and of these only three feelings could be described as 'positive', those of feeling 'safe/secure' (Plutchik *et al.* 1978; Heyman, 1987; Binder and McCoy, 1983), 'happy' (Binder and McCoy, 1983; Heyman, 1987) and 'calm' (Richardson, 1987; Heyman, 1987). The total list of feelings described is shown in Table 11.2 in order of frequency of mention. The selection of the articles was based on the fact that they examined patients' feelings rather than staff's, and many of these were limited in validity.

Every research study examined mentioned anger as being a dominant feeling of patients within seclusion. Despite this no exploration of events has yet taken place to discover why an individual feels angry during seclusion, and whether factors associated with seclusion are contributing to this anger over and above any precursors to the seclusion period.

Nonetheless, it is observed that in studies where both patients and staff were asked if they felt seclusion to be helpful in a general sense, no difference of opinion is found (Hammill *et al.*, 1989). This appears to contradict the feelings described within the literature; however, it may be that such feelings are viewed as a necessary evil, and patients with a low self-esteem may feel that such feelings were deserved in view of their behaviour. It may even be that patients' agreements reflect a sense of 'playing along' with the system, rather than an accurate description of their feelings (Chamberlin, 1985). An interesting study by Richardson (1987) found that 50% of patients felt that seclusion protected them, 40% felt that it protected others, and 58% felt that seclusion was a form of punishment. Even staff were found

Table 11.1 Studies describing feelings of patients in seclusion

Feelings described	1	2	3	4	5	6	7	8	9	10	11	12
Anger	*	*	*	*	*	*	*	*	*	*	*	*
Depression/sadness				*	*	*		*	*	*	*	
Helplessness		*		*	*	*	*	*	*	*	*	
Abandonment				*	*							
Scared/fear		*		*	*	*		*		*	*	*
Worry		*										
Frustration		*									*	*
Boredom	*								*		*	
Confusion	*	*				*			*		*	
Safe/secure		*				*			*			
Disgusted	*					*			*		*	
Trapped/enclosed		*			*							
Imprisoned/punished			*			*	*			*	*	
Resentment											*	*
Humiliation		*				*	*					*
No memory					*							
Felt better										*		
Calm						*				*		
Wound up										*		
Sick										*		
Vindictive										*		
Hurt										*		
Lonely		*							*	*		
Degraded									*			
Dehumanized									*			
Guilt									*			
Relieved						*						
In control						*						
Satisfied						*						
Happy		*				*						
Agitation				*								
Fairly treated		*										
Stimulated		*										
Powerful		*										

Studies used:
1. Binder, 1979.
2. Binder and McCoy, 1983.
3. Chamberlin, 1985.
4. Hammill, 1987.
5. Hammill *et al*, 1989.
6. Heyman, 1987.
7. Jenson, 1985.
8. Norris and Kennedy, 1992.
9. Plutchik *et al*, 1978.
10. Richardson, 1987.
11. Soliday, 1985.
12. Wadeson and Carpenter, 1976.

Table 11.2 Feelings described in 12 available articles

Feelings described by patients	No of articles mentioning feelings described
Anger	12
Helplessness	9
Scared/fear	7
Depression/sadness	7
Imprisoned/punished	5
Confusion	5
Humiliation	4
Disgusted	4
Frustration	3
Abandonment	3
Boredom	3
Lonely	3
Safe/secure	3
Worry	2
Resentment	2
Trapped/enclosed	2
Calm	2
Happy	2
No memory	1
Felt better	1
Wound up	1
Sick	1
Vindictive	1
Hurt	1
Degraded	1
Dehumanized	1
Guilt	1
Relieved	1
In control	1
Satisfied	1
Agitation	1
Fairly treated	1
Stimulated	1
Powerful	1

to believe that seclusion was a form of punishment in a study by Whaley and Ramirez (1980). This again highlights that discrepancies can occur when emotional criteria are examined. It is difficult to be objective about data, but easy to misrepresent and misunderstand what subjects express. It takes a skilled person to 'really know' what another is feeling without having been in a similar situation themselves.

PERCEPTIONS WITHIN SECLUSION

Barradell (1985) found that sensory deprivation occurred within seclusion that led to time perception being altered. However, in a study by Hammill *et al.* (1989), it was felt that time perception was not significantly altered. It would be interesting to evaluate the different procedures within the two institutions studied to assess whether nursing practice differed, which might effect such a change in findings. Hallucinatory experiences have also been described (Van Rybroek *et al.* 1987; Wadeson and Carpenter 1976; Richardson, 1987), and indeed some of the patients found these hallucinations pleasurable. Binder and McCoy's (1983) study found that only four out of 24 patients were able to recall the reason for their seclusion, yet Richardson noted that two out of three of the patients in her study were able to accurately describe why they were secluded. In support of this, Hammill *et al.*, (1989) point out that patients' recollections were 'generally factually accurate except for a tendency in some patients to play down any agitated or aggressive behavior on their part'.

LISTENING TO PATIENTS

As recipients of health services provided for their care, patients' views ought to be held as the most valuable reference tool when providing and evaluating treatment modalities. Mentally ill people are not irrational beings: they are people in need of support as they cope with their own particular problem. Mentally ill people are not to be discredited, even when some aspects of their perception are damaged. We include here some comments from patients interviewed during the course of our research. Hopefully, these will be an accurate representation of the many patients we have seen during our careers. These patients are well worth the time and effort of listening to if services are to adjust and help them most effectively.

Forensic patients' views about seclusion

The following transcripts form a very small fragment of a much larger research study in the use of seclusion within the special hospitals of England and Wales, Ashworth, Broadmoor and Rampton, which at the time of writing is ongoing. In this portion of the study a number (unspecified at present) of patients were interviewed within 7 days of a seclusion experience. The criteria for selection included no previous seclusion experience within a period of 6 months prior to the current seclusion. Part of the interviews involved a semistructured schedule revolving around the three dimensions of time, treatment and efficacy of seclusion. This allowed for a good deal of probing. The interviews were tape-recorded and then transcribed into print. The full SHSA study is due for publication in 1994/5.

Case 1

Interviewer (I) Why were you placed into seclusion in the first instance?

Patient (P) Fighting . . . er . . . with another patient, not with the staff.

I   You started a fight with . . .

P   No, I didn't start it, he did. He wouldn't move and he knew I wanted to clear the tables. I asked him three times to move but he wouldn't. So I whacked him. He was going to hit me so I hit him first. Pre-emptive strike (laugh).

I   Did you walk quietly to the seclusion room?

P   Well, not exactly. The staff had me all twisted up, you know, locks on (control and restraint technique) but I was, er, fighting.

I   And then?

P   Well, when the staff got me to the seclusion room they ripped my clothes off and jabbed me up (injection). But I kept fighting. I didn't give up. They had to scurry out of the room quick.

I   What did you do then?

P   I put my head under the pillow and cried.

I   Why did you put your head under the pillow to cry?

P   I wouldn't let those b******s see me cry.

I   Why were you crying? What were your feelings at that time?

P   I was so frustrated. And I was so angry. And I was so scared. I really hated being put in seclusion. It's really claustrophobic. I can't stand being closed in like that. It's like being treated like an animal. I know I was fighting, but I really hadn't started it and I only hit him because he was going to hit me first. They'd no right doing that to me.

I   What do you think of the way the staff treated you in seclusion?

P   Like dirt. Like its just a job to them. They don't care. They couldn't care less, in fact.

I   Why is that do you think?

P   They think you deserve all you get. They think you deserve to get punished. That's why you're there, for punishment, that's what they think.

I   What did they do to you?

P   Well, nothing really. I mean they didn't ... you know ... beat me up or anything. It's just ... you know they brought me my meals, and a cup of tea, and asked me if I wanted a smoke but ... It's their attitude, they're really detached and couldn't care less. It's that feeling of being entirely alone. Knowing that you are the only one who cares about yourself. So alone. So isolated. The whole world doesn't give a f**k.

I   Did the staffs' attitude change over the period you were in seclusion?

P   They got friendlier. Not with me, but between themselves. Like ... at first when they came in with my meals they wouldn't even talk amongst themselves but as time went on they started cracking jokes between themselves, know what I mean?

I   Yes. Did you know when they were about to terminate the seclusion?

P   Well sort of. They usually let you out the following morning when they came in with breakfast they were friendly – even with me. So I figured the seclusion was about to be stopped.

I   What changes, in you, do you think the staff were looking for before stopping the seclusion?

P   They just want to know if you've learnt your lesson and that you promise not to do it again. Which, of course, you promise. That is if you want to get out, and I did. I hated it in there. It makes you feel totally out of control. They've got all the power.

From this transcript the patient perceives the staff as uncaring,

aloof and distanced. Although it may be the case that the nursing
staff were indeed these things, it may also be the case that they
were not. The patient also perceives the seclusion experience in
negative terms, and suggests that the duration is arbitrarily
linked to 'paying the price'. The sense of isolation and powerlessness are felt very deeply and the seclusion itself is worsened by
the staff's early disregard, as perceived by the patient. The
patient does not indicate that he is aware of any psychiatric
assessment but merely perceives that he has to show some
remorse for his 'offence' and 'promise' not to do it again.

Case 2
Interviewer (I) So, how did you spend the time in seclusion?
Patient (P) I didn't spend it. I lived it. Or perhaps . . . it was more
    like a death. The time did funny things, like . . . stand still.
    And then it would leap by. Sometimes it would go back on
    itself. Sometimes just . . .
I   Were you aware about what time of day it was?
P   Didn't matter.
I   Why?
P   You were locked into your own time in there and there was
    no way out.
I   Did you relate to the time outside of the room?
P   Oh yeah. You always know roughly what time it was in the
    real world 'cos they would bring meals, you know, and get
    you up for a smoke an' that. They'd like come and see you
    at the handover an' check you out. So you knew like it was
    the middle of the day.
I   Did you . . . ?
P   I'll tell you what I did think about. I thought about going
    crazy. At one time I thought my mind had stopped, man. I
    was weird. Like I was dead, or something, and yet I could
    feel the time moving on, slowly.

From this 'snapshot' it can be seen, for this patient, that the time
spent in the seclusion room was reported in similar terms to the
reports in the sensory deprivation studies during the 1950s and
1960s. However, the patient may also have had some element of
psychosis overlay. Notwithstanding, the patient's perception
of time during seclusion was distorted, for one reason or
another.

Case 3

Patient (P) ... I was so angry and humiliated. I had to smile and pretend I was grateful, when all I wanted to do was to get even. They let me go as if they were giving me something. As if it was theirs to give.

Interviewer (I) Did the seclusion help you calm down?

P Christ no, it made me get more and more angry. What it did do was teach me that I had to play the game with them. Let them think I was calmed down.

I Do you think you will end up in seclusion again?

P I hope not ... but ... probably will. Next time though it will be for something worthwhile ... and I'll take at least one of those b******s with me.

I What benefits are there, do you think, in being secluded?

P There's no benefits. It's boring. But what it does do is show people you've still got it. Like you've not given up. They haven't broken you. They may box you (seclusion) but they haven't broken your spirit. You haven't given in.

I What lesson did ...?

P There's no lessons in there, you haven't got time to think about that, you're too busy being angry.

Clearly, the views expressed by this patient would indicate that seclusion was an external control which suppressed behavioural facets, but it is difficult to see whether there is any therapeutic gain in this sense. Although there is no indication that the seclusion was operated as a punitive measure, the patient clearly understands it as a sanction and symbol of status.

Although this study is in its infancy and the chosen transcripts are specific, and as this chapter is concerned about patients' views, we feel the comments stand as worthwhile. At the time of writing, the three cases outlined do reflect the main transcripts.

COMPLAINING ABOUT SECLUSION

Given that seclusion is viewed negatively by patients and that this is often in contrast to the perceptions of nursing staff, it is interesting to observe that very few complaints occur about seclusion practice. This may give the impression that patients accept seclusion practice, but the transcripts and findings discussed earlier clearly demonstrate that patients are often unhappy about it. Indeed, during the course of writing this book, the authors approached agencies to ask their views about seclusion and some declined to be involved because they felt the subject was too painful and sensitive to talk about freely. Because of this it is very difficult to evaluate why this topic is avoided even by those who have experienced seclusion. However, some have put forward their own theories and opinions as to why this should be so.

Reasons for not complaining

A leading barrister points out that the mentally ill are notoriously vulnerable to abuse from their carers. Nonetheless he states that they 'Suffer discrimination in not being allowed to take legal proceedings unless the claim is based on allegations of negligence or bad faith, and even in such cases they must first obtain leave of the High Court, which is withheld unless there is 'substantial ground' for the allegation' (Robertson, 1989). Often complaints made by the mentally ill come down to 'their word against ours', and Jenson (1985) argues that patients do not complain about seclusion because of their realization that they are totally dependent on the staff. The fact that patients know that future care and admissions are dependent on nurses' decisions renders them reluctant to influence that care by complaining about their experience of seclusion. Jenson states that when patients seem accepting of seclusion 'It is not always a positive trend. It expresses more the feeling of complete dependence on the therapists' (Jenson, 1985).

Another explanation, put forward by McElroy (1985) is that 'cognitive dissonance exists among the staff and interferes with their full understanding of the seclusion experience from the patient's perspective'. McElroy goes on to explain that, as this dissonance is uncomfortable, the staff avoid situations that increase it and in doing so, ignore or discount patients' negative views. In this way, any expression of painful experiences made by the patients is rationalized and minimized by the staff, who have to cope with other, more pressing, institutional demands, such as low staffing etc. In this way, it is conceivable that any verbal complaints made by patients (often the first avenue chosen for complaint) are not appreciated by the staff and therefore never examined.

Also, Shields (1985) points out that clinicians are often reluctant to test the effectiveness of treatments if they have advocated these particular approaches. This is a major area of resistance within seclusion practice, and change is slow to alter this so that criticism is seen as helpful rather than abusive. Shields challenges practitioners to examine patients' opinions of services. He concludes: 'We must also ask whether we want to know, and whether we can be flexible enough to admit that the patient may know better than the professional what is best for them' (Shields, 1985). In a later study, Shields points out that patients continue to be passive recipients of care within psychiatry, and that this will remain so until they are allowed more control over their care (Shields *et al.*, 1988). This is extremely important within the seclusion debate, as patients are never given a choice about seclusion and are therefore rendered passive, whether they like it or not.

Complaints and the NHS

In 1990, MIND carried out a survey of mental health service users to discover their feelings about the care they received. They concluded: 'The straightforward message is mental health services can only be effective if they are designed to be sensitive to the needs of people who suffer from, or are vulnerable to, mental distress' (MIND, 1990). One of the main ways to discover the needs of patients is to listen to complaints, and an appropriate avenue for such complaints should be established.

In a more recent paper concerning a general hospital (*Which*, 1993) there are further indications that complaints procedures within the NHS are failing to meet the needs of patients. The report describes NHS procedures as 'bewildering', and found that 41% of complainants at Chase Farm Hospital felt dissatisfied with the way their complaints were handled. Half the patients who complained were dissatisfied with the outcome, yet only one in five of these took their complaint further: the others gave up, expressing helplessness and the fact that they felt it would be a waste of time complaining. Not everyone was told of their right to appeal. It is interesting to note that some of the many reasons for not complaining outlined in the *Which* document include: 'Feeling vulnerable and lacking confidence during illness; feeling grateful for treatment and being reluctant to make a fuss; a fear of victimisation. Even when they are prompted, some people feel they have no right to criticise professionals. Many think it is futile to complain. Others may have difficulty expressing themselves' (*Which*, 1993).

Patients who wish to complain about seclusion are already facing a stigma and lacking confidence due to their illness. If these are reasons put forward not to complain in a general hospital, then they will be all the more powerful in preventing patients complaining within mental health. Also, the fact that there are time limits to making the complaints will prove extremely problematic for the mentally ill, who may not recover as quickly as those in general acute hospitals or services. Often, patients are not even told of their right to complain about treatment, including seclusion, particularly when it is their word against the nurses' that seclusion was necessary. Gostin (1986) tells the story of an individual who complained about ill treatment within a secure unit and had his complaint examined by the very nurses he complained about: not surprisingly, the nurses did not uphold the complaint and the matter was dropped. Patients are already extremely vulnerable, and become more so when they make complaints. Some severely ill people admitted to hospital know they will most probably need to be readmitted at some stage in future, and this can cause problems if they think their complaints are going to result in victimization and criticism by the nursing staff who look after them. This ought to be a consideration in mental health units, as patients who complain can easily become labelled 'troublemakers' and cause nursing staff to be defensive in any future interactions.

In a report compiled by the National Association of Health Authorities and Trusts (NAHAT, 1993), it was pointed out that complaints procedures in the NHS fell drastically short of providing important consumer information when providing health care. The report states: 'The arrangements are seen as being over complex, failing to be user friendly, taking too long, often over defensive and often failing to give any satisfactory explanation for the conclusion reached' (NAHAT, 1993). The consultative paper then outlines proposals to deal with these errors. At the time of publication, however, no definite guidelines have been issued. It remains to be seen how these complaints will be dealt with in the future. However, effecting change in the way the NHS deals with complaints, including a standardization of procedures which is easily understandable and accessible for patients, is vitally important in assessing any treatment or procedures within the organization. Patients have a right to be heard. It is their voice which ultimately indicates that care is meeting their needs appropriately.

12

Conclusions

Ann Alty and Tom Mason

During a visit to Romania in November 1991, one of the authors was invited to assess psychiatric care at an institution in Transylvania. The institution concerned was based at Galda De Jos, high in the mountains, and housed around 350 patients with 130 staff, many of whom were untrained, as Ceaucescu had banned all nurse training during his dictatorship. The director and senior psychiatrist, Dr Baldean, was rightly proud of the work carried out at the institution after the revolution of 1989. Until the west was free to send medicine he had managed his extremely violent patients by using restraints, and felt pleased that appropriate medication had lessened the use of these restraints. Conditions described prior to the revolution were terrible; with no water, drugs or trained staff, Dr Baldean strove to work among the mentally ill sent there from a large catchment area. When asked about the use of seclusion he frowned and shrugged. He did not understand. When asked if he locked patients alone in a cell or room he was aghast. 'We don't do such things here' he explained. 'We don't lock people up when they are upset.' Dr Baldean went on to explain that he had an inner locked area where absconders and extremely violent people were placed together and could be better observed, but no-one was locked up alone – and this in a country purported to have very poor standards of psychiatric care. Dr Baldean also explained that some of his colleagues in other institutions disagreed with his decision. Yet he found that it worked for him and his hospital staff. It was a humbling experience but it highlights the universal difficulty in providing care for the mentally ill. Often it depends on those who have the position and authority to implement such care. These people are often in high management or administrative positions which afford the freedom to offer support and advice to those implementing changes. As Dr Baldean showed his visitors around the wards it was obvious that he was well liked by both his staff and patients. Despite having to overcome major obstacles in caring for the mentally ill, there was still a strong sense of camaraderie and empathy between staff and patients. Obviously, a brief visit cannot provide a complete picture of care provided, but the approach to care was apparent in the interactions and discussions observed. Insofar as Dr Baldean was concerned, he cared for his patients and part of that care included *never* using seclusion.

This book was born of frustration at the lack of knowledge and understanding of the principles and concepts underlying seclusion practice in the 20th century. Mental health nursing has so far failed to ensure that the practice of seclusion is research-based. There are many reasons for this. In Britain it is possible that the combining of nursing qualifications in 1948 (when the National Health Service was established) has severely compromised psychiatric nursing practice. Mental health nursing was a discrete area prior to this date and examinations in practice were established long before those in general nursing. The combination of the two fields has ensured that psychiatric nursing has relied progressively more on the medical model and less on establishing ethical and interactive therapeutic intervention for patients. As Savage (1991) points out: 'If biological problems are demonstrable then a physician, not a psychiatrist should offer treatment'. Unfortunately, biological problems in mental illness are not easily demonstrable and herein lies the crux of the matter.

It is often stated by authors writing on seclusion that the issue is complex, and we would uphold this view because, as we have hopefully demonstrated, decisions and reasoning regarding seclusion have become confused in rhetoric which does little to facilitate clearer understanding. However, locking up a person who continually attacks other people is easy to understand and quite reasonable by common understanding. What has made the issue of seclusion so complex and placed stumbling blocks in the way of any real progress is the medicalization of seclusion itself. Without the rationale of therapy, without the jargon of treatment and without the discourse of medicine the issue would be discussed more appropriately within historical, nursing and sociological perspectives. Once medicine confidently claims to hold the key to understanding such concepts as 'dangerousness' and 'violence', and brings them under the gaze of the medical model, then the assumptions of that model apply. Some of these assumptions include the claim that these concepts can be readily identified, categorized, diagnosed, treated, cured and prognosed. Quite clearly, at this stage of scientific knowledge, the medical model is unsuccessful in dealing with dangerousness and violence, with potentially horrific consequences for the victims.

A major difficulty in establishing official and standardized approaches to seclusion and mental illness is that there is so little useful research available to consider. In the past two decades this has begun to change, but the research so far is piecemeal and has not, until this book, been collated into a comprehensive approach to seclusion practice. The material available highlights major disparities in many areas, including such things as staffing ratios, reasons for seclusion, educative approaches and theoretical constructs. However, because there has been a lack of direct statutory input into seclusion practice since the 1890 Lunacy Act, there is little consensus even in understanding of the term, and even greater difficulty in establishing when seclusion is abusive.

SUMMARY OF PREVIOUS CHAPTERS

Chapter 1 introduced the seclusion debate and its current state of development. It was argued that the emotive discourse used by some authors was generally unhelpful in providing a basis for changing practice. This is not to say that there is not a role for subjectivity within analysis – this book, after all, was born of our subjective opinion that it needed to be written! But unless these emotional claims are based on evidence from research they are merely reduced to points of view, and these points of view are notoriously dismissed. Seclusion, without doubt, falls within the nursing domain, despite all that has been said regarding the multidisciplinary involvement, and unless we tackle the problems encountered in its usage in a professional manner we cannot hope to add credibility to nursing as an inchoate profession. If we are seen by other disciplines to write on the topic in a rudimentary fashion, we will be perceived as professionally immature. This is true for those on all sides of the debate.

In the past there has been a tendency to claim that seclusion has been practised since mental illness was recognized. Unfortunately, we have found no evidence to support this view. In Chapter 2 we located seclusion in historical perspective, dismissing the often cited Soranus as the earliest reference to the use of seclusion. From the primary source it became clear that Soranus did not refer to leaving the patient alone, nor did he instruct the locking of the door. On the contrary, care of the mentally ill was more concerned with calm approaches and soothing massages than isolation and distancing from human contact. It is probably fair to say that the dangerous and violent mentally ill were, indeed, shut away; they may have been locked up in attics, cellars and dungeons for containment or even punitive reasons, but there is no evidence to suggest that this was undertaken for therapy. Indeed, it appears that mental illness was perceived differently within different cultures, and treatments were also dependent on the society and culture of the time. We have, however, found much evidence of restraints being used for the mentally ill. For example, a biblical account found in St Mark's Gospel, Chapter 5 Verse 4, describes a man with 'evil spirits' breaking his chains and leg irons; however, we have not discovered any details which indicate that locking patients alone was considered to be useful. Seclusion as practised today appears to have only arisen as societies 'progressed' and became more organized, and indeed, industrialized. It appears that as western culture developed a need to maintain a status quo within society, so a need to segregate and control those who threatened this arose. There does seem to be a definite trend in this restrictive approach to 'care' for the mentally ill as industrialization developed, which lends support to Scull's (1989) argument.

In Chapter 3 an updated literature review on seclusion was reported which highlighted a diverse approach in attempting to understand further the practice of seclusion. While many studies focus on the associated factors relating to the use of seclusion, others have centred upon the experience of seclusion itself, from both staff and patient perspectives. The literature reviews highlighted the growing concern over the lack of choice regarding alternatives. This is very clearly an area requiring extensive research.

The theoretical underpinning of seclusion use was the theme of Chapter 4, and various conceptual frameworks were drawn together within the 'TCP' schemata. A 'benevolent–malevolent' scale was identified within which the various themes could be located. Although the value of this scale may be limited, it certainly helps towards understanding a diverse and complex issue. The TCP structure is polarized along a continuum which reflects the views from those within the debate.

In Chapter 5 the legal aspects and policy issues were deliberated, beginning with a brief explanation of what must be considered as a major turning point in the review of seclusion: the Boston State case. Seclusion litigation has been, and still is, an issue that is receiving close attention, and without doubt it will feature large in the future. The legal ramifications are centred around human rights and their abuse, but involve complex relationships between victim and perpetrator. Perhaps the fear of such litigation will cause resistance to closer scrutiny of the practice by managers and administrators; however, it would be extremely unhelpful should such legal scrutiny to be forced upon the profession by outside agencies examining such cases as the understanding of human rights infringements gathers momentum. It would surely be more cost-effective to anticipate the moral and legal scrutiny by pre-empting such action and providing a professional forum to debate such issues without the pressure of lawsuits.

Non-seclusion policies and the associated issues were examined and discussed in Chapter 7. It is felt strongly that clinicians and managers have equal responsibility for developing such policies. It has been argued that the establishment of non-seclusion policies needed to be realistic and safe for both staff and patients. It will not suffice for those not working in the clinical area to put others at risk to satisfy their own particular ideal. Those wishing to be ideological ought to lead by example, and ensure that the course they are claiming to be safe is actually so before encouraging others to embark upon it.

The education of psychiatric nurses is also problematic in terms of gaining insight and knowledge about seclusion practice. As the pilot study described in Chapter 8 demonstrates, there is much disagreement among professional lecturers about exactly what is useful and what is not. Some even feel that seclusion is no longer an issue, while others express that it is sadly missing in nurse curricula. It is extremely difficult to know which is the correct view – both seem so certain yet neither agrees. It is obviously a dilemma which is reflected in curriculum choices, and will serve to confuse today's students as much as in the past. Chapter 8 also highlighted the power that nursing bureaucracy plays in maintaining control and stifling innovation. Whistleblowing is examined alongside the role of nurse managers in suppressing it. The fact that complaints by nursing staff regarding seclusion can be dismissed by applying sanctions against the complainants on the grounds of the manner in which the complaint is made is a subtle but crucial point to note. This clearly maintains the nurse, and hence, nursing, in a subservient and submissive position. Project 2000 students are expected to make great headway towards setting higher standards of nursing practice, but such students are very vulnerable in the expectation that they will be able to dismantle extremely powerful, well established and well defended socialization structures in nursing practice. We would argue that this is unfair, and will put unnecessary pressure on nursing students. It is actually the responsibility of the nursing profession as a whole to recognize and work within these structures to improve practice. Placing too much emphasis on the 'educated nurse' rather than the 'trained nurse' will undoubtably cause friction and weaken the professional representation of care given to patients.

In Chapter 9 we explored in detail what we describe as 'seclusion abuse'. We compared the overt, systematic abuse to the more subtle and covert institutional abuse which can create victims within psychiatric structures of care. At this stage we also examined changing seclusion practice and the factors compelling as well as hindering change. Wright (1989) is extremely positive about the ability of nurses to act as agents for change within practice settings. He states: 'The potential to be a change agent lies, to a greater extent, in every nurse' (Wright, 1989).

Change is never easy, but there is certainly a case for changing the nature of seclusion practice even if eradication is not a realistic proposal, and this change will involve organizational and attitudinal factors. It is, perhaps, expecting too much of hurt and injured staff to operate uncomplainingly in a calm, efficient and caring manner whilst nursing those who have caused them their pain. If this is so, then clearly there is a need to address the subtle interpersonal dynamics which can result from such a highly charged emotional atmosphere. We often adopt such terms as political awareness or ethics, and include them within nursing courses in an attempt to give the impression that we are self-aware and bringing nursing into the 1990s. On examination, however, these approaches do not afford a viable means of bringing such concepts and understanding into real-life issues and practice. Clay points out that this gives modern nursing a veneer of respectability, but 'They are not permitted to influence the way nurses behave or to help them towards coping with and dealing with their problems and dilemmas at work' (Clay, 1987). This actually does much damage to pragmatic development, as they become simply words which are used regularly and understood rarely, which inhibits forward development. This was upheld in the pilot study described in Chapter 8. When asked to describe details of subjects taught to preregistration students which were related to seclusion practice, a plethora of words was used, from 'aggression' to 'ethics', with little agreement between the eight nursing colleges as to what was actually valuable content when dealing with seclusion. Sometimes, what we say we are teaching sounds incredibly good and impressive yet has little value in the field of practice. This is why there is much confusion about seclusion practice and why little has yet been agreed at a national level as to its benefits or detriments.

The fact that some continue to feel that all psychiatry is an abuse of the individual (Savage, 1991) implies that many would like to abolish seclusion completely. It is true that seclusion abuse does occur; inquiry reports over the years uphold this fact and when one examines the findings this abuse is horrific. However, most medical and nursing interventions are open to abuse and this does not prevent them being used successfully with careful monitoring and the correct indications. It has been established that seclusion leaves staff with 'unsettled, uncomfortable feelings' (Norris and Kennedy, 1992). As described earlier, these feelings include embarrassment and guilt. It is possible (indeed highly likely) that seclusion has avoided careful scrutiny until recently because of the embarrassment and guilt that may develop when it is used. This is often unfounded, because it has never really been substantiated by true research which indicates valuable approaches to care. The fact that most guidelines state that the procedure should only be used as a 'last resort' may encourage this false guilt, as nurses may feel they have failed when seclusion is finally used.

When analysing seclusion abuse it is important to remember

that aggression and assault are criminal acts. There is a case for re-examining the use of sanctions against those who commit such acts, whether they be committed by staff or patients. In the case of patients there is no recourse in British law for mental patients who assault staff. Such immunity breeds malpractice and makes nurses particularly vulnerable. Being assaulted at work should never be seen as part of the job. Abuse often occurs over a period of time, and there can often be a fine dividing line between abusive intervention and appropriate intervention. Often it is difficult to pinpoint where this line has been breached. It is pointed out that the nurse has a responsibility to 'question the practices of other health care professionals and the policies and functioning of the organizational structure if she feels they are harmful to the patients' (Rumbold, 1986). It has recently been agreed that this is problematic (Tomlin, 1991), yet if change is to occur and questions are to be asked it must be nurses who ask them and influence practice.

In her social audit report on conscientious objectors, Beardshaw (1981) describes the improper use of seclusion as inappropriate custodial patterns of care at Whittingham Hospital, as well as for undue punishment at South Oakden. Beardshaw also describes extreme seclusion abuse at Ely and Winterton. She agrees that any soul-searching about such abuse should come from constructive criticism within the organization itself, and never be forced upon the system by outside agencies. She states: 'But stifling anything that smacks of 'dissent', regardless of the motives that prompt it, means that any hope of self-regulation is generally stillborn. More importantly, such suppression may itself create the conditions in which abuse can become established and continue unnoticed' (Beardshaw, 1981).

Some of this constructive criticism occurs whenever nurses reflect and evaluate their own practice. Ethical reasoning is extremely important in reaching decisions about seclusion practice. In Chapter 10 we identified some of the main underlying ethical principles that should be understood when making decisions about seclusion. So far, little academic rigour has been applied to ethical debate concerning seclusion practice, and this has produced a poor strategy for caring. Nurses do need empirical and scientific knowledge to carry out their work. However, Chinn (1991) rightly points out that this falls short of the total knowledge needed to nurse effectively. Chinn highlights empirics, aesthetics, personal knowledge and ethics as the total knowledge base required and expected of nurses. She states: 'Although empiric knowledge is valuable for nursing practice, each of the patterns of knowing is essential. Each is a distinct aspect of the whole, every pattern makes a contribution to the whole, and each is equally vital' (Chinn, 1991).

There is little ethical discourse surrounding the seclusion debate. In the recent Ashworth Inquiry no-one was invited to discuss ethical issues in relation to seclusion, although there were representatives from the legal profession present. When discussing restraint, Thompson (1992) mentioned in passing that it caused ethical problems for the nurse, but no-one ventured to discuss which ethical problems or principles were involved and conversation quickly reverted to legal matters.

It is true that nursing practice evolves and is never wholly separated from nursing history. As pointed out by Barker and Baldwin (1991): 'Contemporary practice does not exist in a vacuum: we are all part of history and can influence others' history. Our ideas about care, treatment and helping are, at least in part, a function of history. The ideas which shape contemporary practice were themselves once shaped by now out-moded practices' (Barker and Baldwin, 1991).

Seclusion has been handed down through generations of care yet this is not necessarily a reason for unquestioning use of the procedure. Nor does the fact that is an ancient practice mean it has no value today. However, the practice of secluding the adult mentally ill patient needs modern support or discreditation in the form of careful, valid research. Contemporary nursing ethical debate on a national scale would provide a framework in which to link research findings to date. It is from this that appropriate policies and legal constraints may be developed which protect both the patient and nursing staff from abuse.

As ethical understanding involves the values and practices of practitioners, it follows that to build a clearer basis for better understanding of the seclusion issue we need to hear what patients themselves think of the practice. In Chapter 11 we included the feelings and opinions of those who have first-hand knowledge of the practice – the patients. Although there were a few positive comments on seclusion experience, in the main their views are profoundly negative. Patients report anger and helplessness as the predominant feelings while in seclusion, with feelings of humiliation following closely. From the research data presented there appears to be a diverse response from patients, in that they show signs of defiance and non-compliance 'up front' while exhibiting a deep vulnerability hidden within themselves. This vulnerability is often unobserved by the nurses, and will inevitably lead to misunderstandings because at the time nurses too may behave in an off-hand way, which belies their own sense of vulnerability and unease about the practice. This could account for the contradictions discovered within the small amount of existing research into the feelings of patients. Patients may indeed verbalize positive feelings and opinions to the nurses who care for them, and never express their pain due to the simple instinct of surviving and complying in order to have negative sanctions lifted. The sooner they learn to behave the sooner they will go home! Patients' letters and anecdotes declare their feelings on being secluded, against their will and under the control of others.

In an ideal world seclusion would never be used . . . but also in an ideal world no-one would become mentally ill. . . . In no way are we advocating a complete ban on seclusion. We have both used it within our own practice and would never rule out the possibility of using it again should similar situations arise. At present, establishments that use seclusion are ill-equipped to practise alternative strategies, should these exist. The personal safety of both patient and staff is the dominant factor in deciding on seclusion. However, patients who have been secluded view their experience extremely negatively, and this ought to be taken into account when planning care. Neither ought nurses to feel guilt each time they implement seclusion. Provided abuse has not taken place, false guilt is no foundation for changing practice in a helpful way.

In terms of eradicating the use of seclusion, we would argue that eliminating its use for such reasons as 'affronting the dignity of the staff' or the patient being 'noisy' would reduce seclusion use considerably. This is the case for all suggested alternatives. When examined closely, seclusion facilities are maintained because of the explosive violence that can sometimes occur on psychiatric wards, or the fear of staff that such violence may occur. Therefore, if total eradication of seclusion is the objective then clearly the focus of attention should be this core violence. All factors contributing to such violence should come under closer scrutiny, including its origination, diversion, prediction and prevention.

COMMUNITY CARE AND SECLUSION

Attempts have been made to introduce community care in mental health since the 1950s, when the Royal Commission on the Law relating to Mental Illness and Mental Deficiency (1954–57) recommended that there should be a shift from hospital to community care, and this emphasis gathered momentum in the 1960s (Fishwick, 1992). Change has been slow, with numerous papers outlining community care as the ideal, but the most recent effective paper was in 1986, when the Secretary of State for Social Services commissioned a report which examined community care policy. This became known as the 'Griffiths Report' (HMSO, 1988) and led to the National Health Service and Community Care Act 1990. The new Project 2000 courses incorporate this change in approach by focusing care provision within the community. Unfortunately, we fear that concentrating current nursing education on to community issues could lead to problems in seclusion practice. In the pilot study described in Chapter 8, those respondents who felt that seclusion issues were not adequately addressed were invited to comment. The comments were varied, but one is worthy of consideration within this debate as it gives a clear statement as to problems which will be encountered in educating nurses in the future. The point was made that, with nursing becoming more focused on community care, there is little need to teach about seclusion as seclusion always takes place within institutional settings. We hold the view that, while drawing attention to the fact that, where possible, patients are better cared for in their own community environment, the community care approach is not mirrored in inpatient units. We are afraid that this imbalance will be to the detriment of patients who will need inpatient care. As we have discussed, caring within institutions requires an understanding and appreciation of how systems work in order to prevent abuse and mismanagement. This could well be ignored in new nursing approaches, and it is possible that community care will leave such practices as seclusion and restraint within institutions and hidden from view, as all attention is focused upon what goes on outside. It could also transpire that inpatient psychiatric care will be considered as a failure within the community care system, just as seclusion is now considered a failure of the inpatient system, which could lead to inpatient psychiatric care provision being severely compromised and misunderstood. If this is so, it would most certainly be a retrograde step.

FUTURE CONSIDERATIONS

We feel that we have let our patients down very badly by not examining seclusion practice earlier, and that current trends in care of the mentally ill will ignore vital considerations in providing appropriate intervention. There is a certain amount of shame involved in confessing this. Not only personal shame, but shame for the profession of nursing we represent, which has until now been far too concerned with talking about improvements in standards and quality of care and yet somehow missing some of the most fundamental questions which prove we are willing to look at our practice in an adult, non-defensive manner. This is not to say that mental health nursing is useless and valueless: on the contrary, mental health nursing is proving itself invaluable in the care of the mentally ill and we feel that mental health nursing has much to offer modern health care approaches. Yet it must be said that our quest to discover more about seclusion has uncovered far more than we first anticipated. It is true, that in the past decade, units such as Reaside in the Midlands and nurse researchers have uncovered lots of valuable new material and approaches to seclusion, yet we have unearthed considerably more questions than answers and have concluded that there is insufficient evidence on which to base our opinions. This whole area is wide open for would-be researchers to investigate further, and we hope that this book will encourage many others to do so.

There are also many other associated subjects which need further scrutiny alongside seclusion practice in order to give a better overall picture of care. As described in Chapter 1, seclusion is discrete as a method of control, yet it is but one among many. Physical and mechanical restraints as well as chemical restraints all seek to control violent and aggressive behaviour, and need the same fervour of scrutiny by practitioners as does seclusion. Physically restraining someone, euphemistically termed 'gentle holding', in the event of a moderate amount of aggression does not receive the same amount of 'official' scrutiny, despite the increased personal restrictiveness above and beyond that imposed by seclusion; and we are poignantly aware that indignation regarding the use of medication to control patients' behaviour is ominously lacking.

References

Allderidge, P. (1978) Hospitals, madhouses and asylums: cycles in the care of the insane, in *Lectures On The History Of Psychiatry* (eds R.M. Murray and T.H. Turner), Gaskell, London, pp. 28–46.

American Psychiatric Association (1984) *Report of the APA Task Force on the Psychiatric Uses of Seclusion and Restraint*. American Psychiatric Association, Washington.

Angold, A. (1989) Seclusion. *British Journal of Psychiatry,* **154**, 437–44.

Applebaum, P.S. and Guthiel, T.G. (1980) The Boston State Hospital case: 'involuntary mind control', the constitution and 'the right to rot'. *American Journal of Psychiatry,* **137**, 720–23.

Atha, D. (1989) *Report of the Inquiry into the Circumstances Leading to the Death in Broadmoor Hospital of Mr Joseph Watts on 23 August 1988.* SHSA, London.

Atkinson, J. (1991) Autonomy and mental health, in *Ethical Issues In Mental Health* (eds P. Barker and S. Baldwin), Chapman & Hall, London.

Auld, M. (1992) Nurse education past and present. *Nursing Standard,* **6** (22), 37–39.

Bandura, A. (1969) *Principles of Behaviour Modification.* Holt, Rinehart and Winston, London.

Barker, P. and Baldwin, S. (1991) *Ethical Issues In Mental Health,* Chapman & Hall, London.

Barradell, J.G. (1985) Humanistic care of the patient in seclusion. *Journal of Psychosocial Nursing,* **23** (2), 9–15.

Barton, W.E. (1962) *Administration in Psychiatry,* Charles C. Thomas, Springfield Il.

Baudrillard, J. (1983) *Simulations.* Semiotexte, New York.

Baxter, E., Hale, C. and Hafner, R.J. (1989) Use of seclusion in a psychiatric intensive care unit. *Australian Clinical Review,* **9**, 142–45.

Beardshaw, V. (1981) *Conscientious Objectors At Work,* Social Audit, London.

Beauchamp, T. and Childress, J.F. (1983) *Principles Of Biomedical Ethics,* Oxford University Press, New York.

Becker, P. (1986) Advocacy in nursing: perils and possibilities. *Holistic Nursing Practice,* **1** (1), 54–63.

Berlin, R.L. (1975) *Advocacy for Child Mental Health,* Brunner/Mazel, New York.

Binder, R.L. (1979) The use of seclusion on an in-patient crisis intervention unit. *Hospital and Community Psychiatry,* **30** (4), 266–69.

188   *References*

Binder, R.L. and McCoy ,S.M. (1983) Patients' attitudes towards placement in seclusion. *Hospital and Community Psychiatry*, **34**, 1051–54.
Blackburn, M. (1992) Be proud of the project. *Nursing Standard*, **6** (36), 44–45.
Bloch, S. and Reddaway, P. (1977) *Russia's Political Hospitals*, Victor Gollancz, London.
Blom-Cooper, L. (1992) *Report of the Committee of Inquiry into Complaints about Ashworth Hospital*, HMSO, London.
Bourne, L.F., Dominowski, R.L., Loftus, E.F. and Healy, A.F. (1986) *Cognitive Processes*, Prentice Hall, New Jersey.
Brennan, W. (1991) Alone again, naturally. *Nursing Standard*, **6** (7), 46–47.
Brindle, D. (1992) Mental patients terrified by pig's head at 'repressive hospital'. *The Guardian*, 10 March.
Broadhurst, A. (1978) *The Health and Safety at Work Act in Practice*, Heyden, London.
Bronte, C. (1946) *Jane Eyre*, Zodiac Press, London.
Brown, J.S. and Tooke, S.K. (1992) On the seclusion of psychiatric patients. *Journal of Social Science and Medicine*, **35** (5), 711–21.
Burnard, P. and Chapman, C. (1988) Professional and Ethical Issues in *Nursing*, John Wiley, Chichester.
Burrow, S. (1992) The deliberate self harming behaviour of patients within a British special hospital. *Journal of Advanced Nursing*, **17**, 138–148.
Bursten, B. (1975) Using mechanical restraints on acutely disturbed psychiatric patients. *Hospital and Community Psychiatry*, **26**, 757–58.
Campbell, T. (1986) *Human Rights – From Rhetoric to Reality*, Blackwell, London.
Campbell, W., Shepard, H. and Falconer, F. (1982) The use of seclusion. *Nursing Times*, **78** (43), 1821–25.
Carpenter, M.D., Hannon, V.R., McCleery, G. and Wanderling, J.A. (1988) Variations in seclusion and restraint practices by hospital location. *Hospital and Community Psychiatry*, **39** (4), 418–23.
Casey, N. (1992) A rude awakening (Editorial). *Nursing Standard*, **6** (53), 3.
Chamberlain, C. (1992) A qualified failure. *Nursing Standard*, **6** (48), 49.
Chamberlain, J. (1985) An ex-patient's response to Soliday. *Journal of Nervous and Mental Disease*, **173** (5), 288–289.
Chinn, P.L. (1991) *Theory and Nursing: A Systematic Approach*, 3rd edn, Mosby Year Book, London.
Chruszcz, C (1992) *Committee of Inquiry into Complaints About Ashworth Stage II; Seclusion*, HMSO, London.
Clay, T. (1986) Unity for change. *Journal of Advanced Nursing*, **11**, 21–23.
Clay, T. (1987) *Nurses, Power and Politics*, Heinemann, London.
Cohen, S. (1985) *Visions of Social Control: Crime, Punishment and Classification*, Polity Press, Cambridge.
Collins (1982) *Concise English Dictionary*, Collins, London.
Convertino, K., Pinto, R.P. and Fiesta, A.R. (1980) Use of inpatient seclusion at a community mental health centre. *Hospital and Community Psychiatry*, **31** (12), 848–50.

Copeman, W.S.C. (1967) *The Apothecaries 1617–1967*, Pergamon Press, Oxford.

Copp, L.A. (1986) The nurse as advocate for vulnerable persons. *Journal of Advanced Nursing*, **11**, 225–263.

Cormack, D. (1976) *Psychiatric Nursing Observed*, Royal College of Nursing, London.

Craig, C., Ray, F. and Hix, C. (1989) Seclusion and restraint: decreasing the discomfort. *Journal of Psychosocial Nursing and Mental Health Services*, **27** (7), 16–19, 31–32.

Crammer, J. (1990) *Asylum History*, Gaskell, London.

Dabrowski, S., Frydman, L. and Zakowsha-Dabrowski, T. (1986) Physical restraint in Polish psychiatric facilities. *International Journal of Law and Psychiatry*, **8**, 369–82.

Daily Mail, (1985) Storm Over Bid to Free Sex Killer. *Daily Mail* 2 November, 1.

Darley, J.M., Glucksberg, S. and Kinchla, R.A. (1986) *Psychology*, Prentice Hall, New Jersey.

Davidson, N.A., Hemingway, M.J. and Wysoki, T. (1984) Reducing the use of restrictive procedures in a residential facility. *Hospital and Community Psychiatry*, **35** (2), 164–67.

Des Moines Register (1980) 20 Unexplained Deaths Found in Hospital Probe. *Des Moines Register*, 6 August, Iowa.

Dix, D.L. (1843) Address to the Massachusetts Legislature: appeal on behalf of the insane of Massachusetts, in *Documentary History of Psychiatry*, (ed C.E. Goshen), Vision Press, London, 1967, pp. 502–4.

Downie, R.S. and Calman, K.C. (1987) *Healthy Respect*, Faber & Faber, London.

Dyer, C. (1991) Pindown Payments Could Top £2m. *The Guardian*, 9 August.

Einhorn, H.J. and Hogarth, R.M. (1981) Behavioural decision theory: processes of judgement and choice. *Annual Review of Psychology*, **32**, 53–88.

Farmer, B. (1993) The use and abuse of power in nursing. *Nursing Standard*, **7** (23), 33–36.

Fernando, S. (1988) *Race and Culture in Psychiatry*, Croom Helm, London.

Fernando, S. (1991) *Mental Health, Race and Culture*, Macmillan, London.

Fishwick, C. (1992) *Community Care and Control*, Pepar, Birmingham.

Fitzgerald, R.G. and Long, I. (1973) Seclusion in the treatment and management of severely disturbed manic and depressed patients. *Perspectives in Psychiatric Care*, **11**, 59–64.

Flaherty, J.A. and Meagher, R. (1980) Measuring racial bias in inpatient treatment. *American Journal of Psychiatry*, **137** (6), 679–82.

Ford, C. and Jones, C. (1992) Students' perceptions of Project 2000. *Nursing Standard*, **6** (6), 30–32.

Foucault, M. (1967) *Madness and Civilisation: A History of Insanity in the Age of Reason*, Tavistock, London.

Foucault, M. (1980) *Power/Knowledge: Selected Interviews and Other Writings 1972–77*. Harvester Press, London.

Foucault, M. (1988) *Politics, Philosophy, Culture: Interviews and Other Writings 1977–84*, Routledge, London.

Francis, E. (1985) How did Michael Dean Martin die? *Open Mind*, **13**, Feb/Mar.

Freedman, S. and Greenblatt, M. (1960) Studies in isolation: hallucinations and other cognitive findings. *United States Armed Forces Medical Journal*, **11**, 1479–97.

Gair, D.S. (1980) Limit-setting and seclusion in the psychiatric hospital. *Psychiatric Opinion*, **17**, 15–19.

Gair, D.S. (1984) Guidelines for children and adolescents, in *The Psychiatric Uses of Seclusion and Restraint*, (ed K. Tardiff), American Psychiatric Press, Washington DC, pp. 69–86.

Gallego, A.P. (1983) *Evaluating the School*, Royal College of Nursing, London.

Gentilin, J. (1987) Room restriction: a therapeutic prescription. *Journal of Psychosocial Nursing*, **25** (7), 12–16.

Gerlock, A. and Solomons, H.C. (1983) Factors associated with the seclusion of psychiatric patients. *Perspectives in Psychiatric Care*, **21** (2), 47–53.

Gibson, B. (1989) The use of seclusion. *Nursing*, **3** (43), 24–26.

Glover, M. (1984) *The Retreat, York*, William Sessions, London.

Goffman, E. (1963) *Stigma*, Prentice Hall, New York.

Goffman, E. (1968) *Asylums: Essays on the Social Situation of Mental Patients and Other Inmates*, Pelican Books, London.

Goshen, C.E. (1967) *Documentary History of Psychiatry*, Vision Press, London.

Gostin, L. (1983) *A Practical Guide to Mental Health Law*, London, MIND.

Gostin, L. (1986) *Institutions Observed*, King Edward's Hospital Fund For London, London.

Grassian, S. and Friedman, N. (1986) Effects of sensory deprivation in psychiatric seclusion and solitary confinement. *International Journal of Law and Psychiatry*, **8**, 49–65.

Greenblatt, M. (1980) Seclusion as a means of restraint. *Psychiatric Opinion*, **17**, 13–14.

Griesinger, W. (1845) Pathology and therapy of psychiatric illness, in *Documentary History of Psychiatry*, (ed C.E. Goshen), Vision Press, London, 1967, pp. 385–417.

Grigson, J.W. (1984) Beyond patient management: the therapeutic use of seclusion and restraints. *Perspectives in Psychiatric Care*, **22** (4), 137–42.

Gutheil, T.G. (1978) Observations on the theoretical bases for seclusion of the psychiatric in-patient. *American Journal of Psychiatry*, **135** (3), 325–328.

Gutheil, T.G. (1980) Restraint versus treatment: seclusion as discussed in the Boston State case. *American Journal of Psychiatry*, **137**, 718–19.

Gutheil, T. G.and Tardiff, K. (1984) Indications and contraindications for seclusion and restraint, in *The Psychiatric Uses of Seclusion*, (ed K. Tardiff), American Psychiatric Press Washington, pp. 11–18.

Hafner, R.J., Lammersma, J., Ferris, R. and Cameron, M. (1989) The use of seclusion: a comparison of two psychiatric intensive care units. *Australian and New Zealand Journal of Psychiatry*, **23**, 235–39.

Hammill, K. (1987) Seclusion: inside looking out. *Nursing Times*, **83** (5), 38–39

Hammill, K., McEvoy, J., Koral, H. and Schneider, N. (1989) Hospitalized schizophrenic patient views about seclusion. *Journal of Clinical Psychiatry*, **83** (5), 38–39.

Harris, A. (1957) Sensory deprivation and schizophrenia. *Journal of Mental Sciences*, **105**, 235–37.

Heyman, E. (1987) Seclusion. *Journal of Psychosocial Nursing and Mental Health Services*, **25** (11), 8–12, 35, 37.

HMSO (1959) *Mental Health Act*, HMSO, London.

HMSO (1967) *Criminal Law Act*, HMSO, London.

HMSO (1974) *Health and Safety at Work Act*, HMSO, London.

HMSO (1980) *Report of the Review of Rampton Hospital*, HMSO, London.

HMSO (1983) *Mental Health Act 1983*, HMSO, London.

HMSO (1984) *Human Rights in the United Kingdom*, HMSO, London.

HMSO (1988) *Community Care: Agenda for Action*, HMSO, London.

HMSO (1990) *Mental Health Act Commission: Code of Practice*, HMSO, London.

HMSO (1992) *Patients' Charter*, HMSO, London.

Hodgkinson, P. (1985) The use of seclusion. *Journal of Medicine, Science and the Law*, **25** (3), 215–22.

Irwin, M. (1987) Are seclusion rooms needed on child psychiatric units? *American Journal of Orthopsychiatry*, **57** (1), 125–26.

Ishiyama, T. and Hewitt, E.B. (1966) Seclusion: a lesson for aides. *Journal of Psychiatric Nursing*, **4**, 563–70.

Jacobs, F.G. (1975) *The European Convention on Human Rights*, Clarendon Press, Oxford.

Jenson, K. (1985) Comments on Dr Stanley M. Soliday's 'A Comparison of Patient and Staff Attitudes Towards Seclusion'. *Journal of Nervous and Mental Disease*, **173**, 290–291.

Jones, E.W. (1982) Advocacy – a tool for radical nursing curriculum planners. *Journal of Nursing Education*, **21** (1), 40–45.

Jones, G., Janman, K., Payne, R. and Rick, T. (1987) Some determinants of stress in psychiatric nurses. *International Journal of Nursing Studies*, **24** (2), 129–44.

Jones, K. (1955) *Lunacy, Law and Conscience*, Routledge & Kegan Paul, London.

Jones, K. (1960) *Mental Health And Social Policy 1845–1959*, Routledge & Kegan Paul, New York.

Jorsh, M. (1991) Transcultural psychiatry. *Postgraduate Update*, 15 September, 360–63.

Keith, C. (1984) *The Aggressive Adolescent*, Free Press, New York.

Kellner, D. (1989) *Jean Baudrillard: from Marxism to Postmodernism and Beyond*, Polity Press, Cambridge.

Kendrick, K. (1991) A baseline for practice. *Nursing*, **4**, 34.

Kendrick, K. and Simpson, A. (1992) The nurses' reformation: philosophy and pragmatics of Project 2000, in *Themes and Perspectives in*

Nursing, (eds K. Soothill, C. Henry and K. Kendrick), Chapman & Hall, London, pp. 91–100.

Kilgalen, R.K. (1977) The effective use of seclusion. *Journal of Psychiatric Nursing and Mental Health Service*, **15** (1), 22–25.

Kingdon, D.G. and Bakewell, E.W. (1988) Aggressive behaviour: evaluation of a non-seclusion policy of a district psychiatric service. *British Journal of Psychiatry*, **153**, 631–34.

Kirkbride, T. (1854) On the construction, organisation and general arrangements of hospitals for the insane, in *Documentary History of Psychiatry*, (ed C.E. Goshen), Vision Press, London, 1967, pp. 505–26.

Kirkpatrick, H. (1989) A descriptive study of seclusion: the unit environment, patient behaviour and nursing interventions. *Archives of Psychiatric Nursing*, **3** (1), 3–9.

Kohnke, M. (1980) The nurse as advocate. *American Journal of Nursing*, November, 2038–40.

Komrad, M.S. (1983) A defence of medical paternalism. Maximising patients' autonomy. *Journal Of Medical Ethics*, **9**, 38–44.

Krause, E.A. (1977) *Power and Illness: the Political Sociology of Health and Medical Care*, Elsevier, New York.

Laing, R.D. (1982) *The Voice of Experience*, Allen Lane, London.

Laing, R.D. (1985) *Wisdom, Madness and Folly*, Macmillan, London.

Lancaster, W. (1982) Health care marketing: a model for planning change, in *The Nurse As Change Agent*, (eds J. Lancaster and W. Lancaster), CV Mosby, St Louis, pp. 344–361.

Lawson, W.B., Yesavage, J.A. and Werner, P.D. (1984) Race, violence, and psychopathology. *Journal of Clinical Psychiatry*, **45** (7), 294–97.

Leff, J. (1988) *Psychiatry Around the Globe: A Transcultural View*, 2nd Edn, Gaskell, London.

Leopoldt, H. (1985) A secure and secluded spot . . . seclusion of patients in psychiatric hospitals. *Nursing Times*, **81** (6), 26–28.

Levi-Strauss, C. (1962) *Totemism*, Merlin Press, London.

Linkenhoker, D.D. (1974) Increasing the effectiveness of time-out from reinforcement. *Psychotherapy: Theory, Research and Practice*, **11**, 326–28.

Linton, M. (1991) Disturbed child centre to close after drug ban. *The Guardian*, 26 June, p. 2.

Lion, J.R., Snyder, W. and Merrill, G.L. (1981) Underreporting of assaults on staff in a state hospital. *Hospital and Community Psychiatry*, **32** (7), 497–98.

Lovaas, O.I., Freitas, L., Nelson, K. and Whalen, C. (1974) Perspectives in behaviour modification with deviant children, in *The Establishment of Imitation and Its Use for the Development of Complex Behaviour in Schizophrenic Children*, (eds O.I. Lovaas and B.D. Bucher), Prentice Hall, New Jersey.

Lowry, M. (1992) Preventing P2000 Chaos. *Nursing Standard*, **6** (28), 46–47.

McCoy, S.M. and Garritson, S. (1983) Seclusion, the process of intervening. *Journal of Psychosocial Nursing and Mental Health Services*, **21** (8), 6–15.

Macdonald, A. (1988) Changing professional practice. *Senior Nurse*, **8** (11), 4–7.

Macdonald, A. (1989) Reducing seclusion in a psychiatric hospital. *Nursing Times*, **85** (23), 58–59.

Macdonald, M. (1980) Insanity and the realities of history in early modern England, in *Lectures on the History of Psychiatry* (ed R.M. Murray and T.H. Turner), Gaskell, London.

McElroy, E. (1985) Consumers of psychiatric services and staff. *Journal of Nervous and Mental Disease*, **73** (5), 287.

McGovern, T.F. (1991) Forward in ethical issues, in *Mental Health*, (eds P. Barker and S. Baldwin), Chapman & Hall, London, pp. xiv–xvi.

Maddison, D., Day, P. and Leabeater, B. (1975) *Psychiatric Nursing*, Churchill Livingstone, Edinburgh.

Mason, T. (1989) *The Decision Making Process in the Initiation of a Seclusion Regime in a Special Hospital*, Unpublished BSc Thesis, Manchester Polytechnic.

Mason, T. (1991) *Seclusion: a Literature Review*, Special Hospitals Service Authority, London.

Mason, T. (1992) Seclusion: definitional interpretations. *Journal of Forensic Psychiatry*, **3** (2), 261–70.

Mason, T. (1993a) Seclusion theory reviewed: a benevolent or malevolent intervention. *Journal of Medicine, Science and the Law*, **33** (2), 95–102.

Mason, T. (1993b) Seclusion: international comparisons. *Journal of Medicine, Science and the Law*, (in Press).

Mason, T. and Chandley, M. (1990) Nursing models in a special hospital: a critical analysis of efficacy. *Journal of Advanced Nursing*, **15**, 667–73.

Mattson, M.R. and Sacks, M.H. (1978) Seclusion: uses and complications. *American Journal of Psychiatry*, **135**, 1210–13.

Mendel, W. and Green, G.(1967) *The Therapeutic Management of Psychological Illness*, Basic Books, New York.

Mill, J.S. (1962) On liberty, in *Utilitarianism*, (ed M. Warnock), Collins, London.

Millar, B. (1991) I have in my hand a piece of paper. *Health Service Journal*, November, p. 12.

Miller, R. (1992) Seclusion: a last sanctuary? *Nursing Standard*, **6** (30), 44–45.

Mills, M.J. (1981) The continuing clinicolegal conundrum of the Boston State Hospital case. *Medico-Legal News*, **9**, 9–18.

MIND (undated) *Being Informed And Giving Consent – A Checklist for Users Of Mental Health Services*. Putting People First Information Leaflet, MIND, London.

MIND (1990) *People First*, MIND, London.

MIND (1991) *Policy On User Involvement*, MIND, London.

Morrison, E.F. (1990a) The tradition of toughness: a study of nonprofessional nursing care in psychiatric settings. *Image: Journal of Nursing Scholarship*, **22** (1), 32–38.

Morrison, E.F. (1990b) Violent psychiatric inpatients in a public hospital. *Scholarly Inquiry for Nursing Practice: An International Journal*, **4** (1), 65–82.

Morrison, P. (1990) A multidimensional scalogram analysis of the use of seclusion in acute psychiatric settings. *Journal of Advanced Nursing,* **15** (1), 59–66.

Morrison, P. and le Roux, B. (1987) The practice of seclusion. *Nursing Times* (Occasional Paper), **83**, 19.

Moss, A.R. (1988) Determinants of patient care: nursing process or nursing attitudes? *Journal Of Advanced Nursing,* **13**, 615–20.

Myers, S. (1990) Seclusion: a last resort measure. *Perspectives in Psychiatric Care,* **26**, 3.

NAHAT (1993) *Complaints Do Matter,* NAHAT, London.

Naish, J. (1992) Discipline. *Nursing Standard,* **7** (1), 20–21.

Nelson, S.H., McKinney. A., Ludwig, K. and Davis, R. (1983) An unusual death of a patient in seclusion. *Hospital and Community Psychiatry,* **34**, 3.

Norris, M.K. and Kennedy, C.W. (1992) How patients perceive the seclusion process. *Journal of Psychosocial Nursing,* **30** (3), 7.

O'Brien, A. (1989) Seclusion. *NSNA Imprint,* November, 79–80.

Oldham, J.M., Russakoff, L.M. and Prusnofsky, L. (1983) Seclusion: patterns and milieu. *Journal of Nervous and Mental Disease,* **171** (11), 645–50.

Outlaw, F. and Lowery, B.J. (1992) Seclusion – the nursing challenge. *Journal of Psychosocial Nursing,* **30**, 4.

Owen, G.M. (1988) For better for worse: nursing in higher education. *Journal of Advanced Nursing,* **13**, 3–13.

Packard, E. (1885) Modern persecution, or insane asylums unveiled, in *Documentary History of Psychiatry,* (ed C.E. Goshen), Vision Press, London, 1967, pp. 640–65.

Parsons, T. (1951) *The Social System,* Routledge and Kegan Paul, London.

Pearson, A. and Vaughan, B. (1986) *Nursing Models For Practice,* Heinemann, Oxford.

Philips, P. and Nasr, S.J. (1983) Seclusion and restraint and prediction of violence. *American Journal of Psychiatry,* **140** (2), 229–232.

Pilette, P.C. (1978) The tyranny of seclusion: a brief essay. *Journal of Psychiatric Nursing,* **16** (10), 19–21.

Pinel, P. (1806) Treatise on mental alienation, in *Documentary History of Psychiatry,* (ed C.E. Goshen), Vision Press, London, 1967, pp. 257–65.

Pink, G. (1993) Whistle down the drain. *Nursing Standard,* **7** (17), 47.

Plutchik, R., Karasu, T.B., Conte, H.R., Siegal, B. and Jerret, I. (1978) Toward a rationale for the seclusion process. *Journal of Nervous and Mental Disease,* **166** (8), 571–79.

Porter, S. (1992) Institutional restraints upon educational reforms: the case of mental health nursing. *Nurse Education Today,* **12**, 452–57.

Powell, D. (1982) *Learning To Relate,* Royal College of Nursing, London.

Price, B. (1985) Your move nurse. *Nursing Times,* 2 October, pp. 24–26.

Ramchandani, D., Akhtar, S. and Helfrich, J. (1981) Seclusion of psychiatric in-patients: a general hospital perspective. *International Journal of Social Psychiatry,* **27** (4), 309–15.

Raz, J. (1986) *The Morality Of Freedom,* Oxford University Press, Oxford.

Redmond, F.C. (1980) Study on the use of seclusion. *Quality Review Bulletin,* **6** (8), 20–23.

Rendon, D., Davis, K. *et al.* (1986) The right to know. The right to be taught. *Journal of Gerontological Nursing*, **12** (12), 33.

Richardson, B.K. (1987) Psychiatric inpatients perceptions of the seclusion room experience. *Nursing Research*, **36** (4), 234–38.

Richman, J. and Mason, T. (1992) Quo vadis the special hospitals?, in *Private Risks and Public Dangers*, (eds S. Scott, G. Williams, S. Platt and H. Thomas), Aldershot, Avebury, pp. 150–67.

Ritchie, S. (1985) *Report to the Secretary of State for Social Services Concerning the Death of Mr Michael Martin at Broadmoor Hospital on 6 July 1984*, HMSO, London.

Ritter, S. (1989) *Manual of Clinical Psychiatric Nursing. Principles and Procedures*, Harper & Row, London.

Robb, B. (1967) *Sans Everything*, Nelson, London.

Robertson, G. (1989) *Freedom, the Individual and the Law*, 6th edn, Penguin, London.

Rolfe, G. (1990) The assessment of therapeutic attitudes in the psychiatric setting. *Journal of Advanced Nursing*, **15**, 564–70.

Roper, J.M., Coutts, A., Sather, J. and Taylor, R. (1985) Restraint and seclusion: a standard and standard care plan. *Journal of Psychosocial Nursing*, **23** (6), 18–23.

Rosen, G. (1968) *Madness In Society*, Routledge & Kegan Paul, London.

Rosen, H. and DiGiacomo, J.W. (1978) The role of physical restraint in the treatment of psychiatric illness. *Journal of Clinical Psychiatry*, **39** (3), 228–33.

Roth, L., Meisel, A. and Lidz, C. (1983) Tests of competency to consent to treatment, in *Medical Ethics*, (eds N. Abrams and M. Buckner), Massachusetts Institute Of Technology, Cambridge, MA.

Royal College of Nursing. Society of Psychiatric Nurses (1979) *Seclusion and Restraint in Hospitals and Units for the Mentally Disordered*, RCN, London.

Royal College of Nursing (1985) *Education Of Nurses: A New Dispensation*, RCN, London.

Royal College of Nursing (1992) *Seclusion Control and Restraint*, RCN, London.

Royal College of Psychiatrists (1981) Isolation of patients in protected rooms during psychiatric treatment. *Bulletin*, **5**, 96.

Royal College of Psychiatrists (1982) Locking up patients by themselves. *Bulletin*, **6**, 199–200.

Royal College of Psychiatrists (1990) The seclusion of psychiatric patients. *Psychiatric Bulletin*, **14**, 500–501.

Rumbold, G. (1986) *Ethics in Nursing Practice*, Bailliere Tindall, London.

Rush, B. (1810) Letter to the managers of the Pennsylvania Hospital, in *Documentary History of Psychiatry*, (ed C.E. Goshen), Vision Press, London, 1967, pp. 281–4.

Russell, D., Hodgkinson, P. and Hillis, T. (1986) Time out. *Nursing Times*, 26 February, 47.

Sallah, D. (1992) Points of view: seclusion. *Nursing Standard*, **6** (21), 43.

Salvage, J. (1985) *The Politics Of Nursing*, Heinemann, London.

Salvage, J. (1988) Professionalization – or struggle for survival? A consideration of current proposals for the reform of nursing in the United Kingdom. *Journal of Advanced Nursing*, **13**, 515–19.

Savage, J. (1987) *Nurses, Gender and Sexuality*, Heinemann, London.

Savage, P. (1991) Abuse by psychiatry. *Senior Nurse*, **11** (5), 36.

Schipperheijn, L.A. and Dunne, F. (1991) Managing violence in psychiatric hospitals. *British Medical Journal*, **303**, 71–72.

Schmied, K. and Ernst, K. (1983) Isolierung und Zwangsinjektion im Urteil der betroffenen Patienten und des Pflegepersonals (Seclusion and emergency sedation: opinions of patients and nursing staff). *Archiv fur Psychiatrik Nervenkrest*, **233**, 211–22.

Schutz, A. (1970) *On Phenomenology and Social Relations*, University of Chicago Press, Chicago.

Schwab, P.J. and Lahmeye, C.B. (1979) The uses of seclusion on a general hospital psychiatric unit. *Journal of Clinical Psychiatry*, **40**, 228–31.

Scull, A. (1989) *Social Order/Mental Disorder*, Routledge, London.

Seedhouse, D. (1986) *Health – the Foundations For Achievement*, Wiley, Chichester.

Seedhouse, D. (1988) *Ethics – the Heart of Health Care*, Wiley, Chichester.

Seguin, E. (1866) Moral treatment, in *Documentary History of Psychiatry*, (ed C.E. Goshen), Vision Press, London, 1967, pp. 165–78.

Seligman, M. (1975) *Helplessness – on Depression, Development and Death*, W.H. Freeman, San Fransisco.

Shields, P. (1985) The consumer's view of psychiatry. *Hospital and Health Services Review*, May, 117–19.

Shields, P., Morrison, P. and Hart, D. (1988) Consumer satisfaction on a psychiatric ward. *Journal of Advanced Nursing*, **13**, 396–400.

Sim, M. and Gordon, E.B. (1972) *Basic Psychiatry*, 2nd edn, Churchill Livingstone, Edinburgh.

Simpson, I.H. (1979) *From Student To Nurse*, Cambridge University Press, Cambridge.

Singer, P. (1979) *Practical Ethics*, Oxford University Press, Oxford.

Soliday, S.M. (1985) A comparison of patient and staff attitudes towards seclusion. *Journal of Nervous and Mental Disease*, **173** (5), 282–86.

Soloff, P.H. (1978) Behavioural precipitants of restraint in the modern milieu. *Comprehensive Psychiatry*, **19**, 179–84.

Soloff, P.H. (1987) Physical controls: the use of seclusion and restraint in modern psychiatric practice, in *Clinical Treatment and Management of the Violent Person*, (ed L.H. Roth), Guildford Press, London, pp. 119–37.

Soloff, P.H. and Turner, S.M. (1981) Patterns of seclusion. *Journal of Nervous and Mental Disease*, **169** (1), 37–44.

Soloff, P.H., Gutheil, T.G. and Wexlet, D.B. (1985) Seclusion and restraint in 1985: a review and update. *Hospital and Community Psychiatry*, **36** (6), 652–57.

Soranus of Ephesus, Caelius Aurelianus (5?? AD) Madness or insanity, in *Documentary History of Psychiatry*, (ed C.E. Goshen), Vision Press, London, 1967, pp. 18–32.

Sparkes, A.W. (1991) *Understanding Philosophy: A Wordbook*, Routledge, London/New York.

Sreenivasan, U. (1983) Limitation of freedom of movement in adult psychiatric units. *Canadian Journal of Psychiatry*, **28** (1), 64–67.

Stein, T. (1993) A voice in the wilderness. *Health Service Journal*, 4 March, 30–31.

Stilling, L. (1992) The pros and cons of physical restraints and social control. *Journal of Psychosocial Nursing*, **30** (3), 1629–33.

Stover, E. and Nightingale, E. (1985) *The Breaking of Bodies and Minds*, Freeman, New York.

Strutt, R., Bailey, C., Peermohamed, R., Forrest, A.J. and Corton, B. (1980) Seclusion: can it be justified? *Nursing Times*, **76**, 1629–33.

Sun (1989) Monster in Shop Trip Horror. *Sun*, 22 February, 1.

Sutor, J.A. (1993) Can nurses be effective advocates? *Nursing Standard*, **7** (22), 30–32.

Szasz, T. (1962) *The Myth of Mental Illness*, Granada, London.

Szasz, T. (1973) *Ideology and Insanity*, Calder and Boyars, London.

Szasz, T. (1974) *Law, Liberty and Psychiatry*, Routledge & Kegan Paul, London.

Szasz, T. (1978) The case against compulsory interventions. *Lancet*, **1**, 1035–36.

Szasz, T. (1983) *Ideology and Insanity*, Marion Boyars, London.

Tardiff, K. (1981) Emergency measures for psychiatric inpatients. *Journal of Nervous and Mental Disease*, **169**, 614–18.

Tardiff, K. (1984) Characteristics of assaultive patients in private hospitals. *American Journal of Psychiatry*, **141** (10), 1232–35.

Teasdale, K. (1987) Stigma and psychiatric day care. *Journal of Advanced Nursing*, **12**, 339–346.

Thomas, P. (1988) Managing change. *Nursing Times*, **84** (44), 58.

Thompson, P. (1986) The use of seclusion in psychiatric hospitals in the Newcastle area. *British Journal of Psychiatry*, **149**, 471–74.

Thompson, P. (1987) Trends in seclusion practice in the Newcastle area. *Bulletin of the Royal College of Psychiatrists*, **2**, 82–84.

Thompson, T. (1992) *Committee of Inquiry into Complaints About Ashworth Hospital. Stage II Transcripts*, 5 March, HMSO, London.

Thorpe, J.G. (1980) Time-out or seclusion? *Nursing Times*, **76** (14), 604.

Tomlin, Z. (1991) Whistling down the wind. *Health Service Journal*, 12 December, 14.

Tooke, S.K. and Brown, J.S. (1992) Seclusion on a psychiatric unit: a comparison of patient and staff perceptions. *Journal of Psychosocial Nursing*, **30** (8), 23–26.

United Kingdom Central Council (1984) *Code Of Professional Conduct*, UKCC, London.

United Kingdom Central Council (1986) *Project 2000 – A New Preparation For Practice*, UKCC, London.

United Kingdom Central Council (1992a) *Code Of Professional Conduct*, UKCC, London.

United Kingdom Central Council (1992b) *The Scope Of Professional Practice*, UKCC, London.

Van Rybroek, G., Kuhlman, T., Maier, G. and Kaye, M. (1987) Preventive aggression devices: ambulatory restraints as an alternative to seclusion. *Journal of Clinical Psychiatry,* **48** (10), 401–4.

Wadeson, H. and Carpenter, W.T. (1976) Impact of the seclusion room experience. *Journal of Nervous and Mental Disease,* **163**, 318–28.

Wagg, B. and Yurick, A. (1983) Care enough to hear. *Journal of Gerontological Nursing,* **9**, 9.

Way, B.B. (1986) The use of restraint and seclusion in New York State psychiatric centers. *International Journal of Law and Psychiatry,* **8**, 383–93.

Way, B.B. and Banks, S.M. (1990) Use of seclusion and restraint in public psychiatric hospitals: patient characteristics and facility effects. *Hospital and Community Psychiatry,* **41** (1), 75–81.

Webster, G.A. (1990) Nursing and the philosophy of science, in *Current Issues In Nursing,* 3rd edn, (ed J.C. McCloskey and H.K. Grace), CV Mosby, Missouri, pp. 12–16.

Wells, D.A. (1972) The use of seclusion on a university hospital psychiatric floor. *Archives of General Psychiatry,* **26**, 410–13.

Westermeyer, J. and Kroll, J. (1978) Violence and mental illness in a peasant society: characteristics of violent behaviours and 'folk' use of restraint. *British Journal of Psychiatry,* **133**, 529–41.

Wexler, D.B. (1982) Seclusion and restraint: lessons from law, psychiatry and psychology. *International Journal of Law and Psychiatry ,* **5**, 285–94.

Whaley, M.S. and Ramirez, L.F. (1980) The use of seclusion rooms and physical restraints in the treatment of psychiatric patients. *Journal of Psychiatric Nursing and Mental Health Services,* **18**, 13–16.

WHICH (1993) Complaining to the NHS. *WHICH,* April, 11–15.

White, R. (1985) Political regulators in British nursing, in *Political Issues In Nursing: Past Present and Future,* (ed R. White), John Wiley, Chichester.

Witts, P. (1992) Patient advocacy in nursing, in *Themes and Perspectives in Nursing,* (ed K. Soothill, K. Kendrick and C. Henry), Chapman & Hall, London, pp. 158–79.

World Health Organization (1982) *Nurses in Support of the Goal of Health For All by the Year 2000,* WHO, Geneva.

World Health Organization (1984) *Education and Training of Nurse Teachers and Managers With Special Regard to Primary Health Care,* WHO, Geneva.

Wright, S.G. (1989) *Changing Nursing Practice,* Edward Arnold, London.

Wulff, H., Pederson, S. and Rosenberg, R. (1990) *Philosophy Of Medicine,* 2nd Edn, Blackwell, London.

Zeidler-Kornmann *v* Federal Republic of Germany. *Yearbook 11* (p. 1020).

Index

English National Board 139
Ethics 110, 115, 120, 146–60
European convention on human
   rights 80–81
Evangelicalism 23
External/internal control 53, 58,
   169
Eyre, Jane 21

Family 84, 127, 131
Fear 1, 13, 20, 59, 78, 100, 101, 106,
   108
Feelings (in seclusion) 46, 100,
   127, 134, 156, 157, 161–73
Forensic nursing, patients,
   psychiatry 6, 27–8, 64, 84,
   128, 166–9
Freedom 48, 68, 69, 104, 174

Gaskell, Dr Samuel 25
General Nursing Council 29, 75
George III 23
Guidelines (for practice) 73, 74,
   76, 77, 78, 81, 119, 147
Guilt 57, 138, 147

Health and Safety at Work
   Act 77–8
Helplessness 137, 156–7, 171
Holism 124
Hypnotic 28

Institution 1, 18, 82–6, 130–32

Labelling 114, 130
Lancaster Moor 25
Law 16, 21–5, 31, 65–81
Legal 65–81
Liberty 153
Lord Eldon 24
Lord Shaftsbury 25
Lunacy Act 1890 28

Machoism 98, 136
Madhouses 18, 22–4
Madhouses Act 31
Management 14, 22, 37, 74, 77–8,
   95–109
Manchester Lunatic Hospital 23

Maximum security 36, 91
Medical model 100, 115, 143, 148,
   175
Medicalization 175
Medication 8, 9, 13, 28–9, 36,
   39, 51, 53, 66–8, 79, 86,
   96–7, 99–100, 106, 109, 138,
   150, 152, 157, 174, 186
Mental health 1, 3, 10, 12, 28, 33,
   71, 97, 110, 114, 125, 126, 127,
   141
Mental Health Act 1959; 1983 29,
   31, 74, 76, 83
Mental Health Act
   Commission 96
Mentally handicapped,
   disordered 73, 154
MIND 29, 121, 171

National Health Service 175
National Health Services Act 31
Neglect 25, 116, 119, 127
Non-maleficence 149, 156–7
Norms 90, 113, 135, 141, 150, 154
Nurse education 15, 110–26
Nurse training 75, 110–26, 144,
   174
Nursing
   care 8, 13, 85, 96
   staff 47, 58–60, 64, 69, 85–7
   theory 113

Objective 64, 105–8, 130
Observations 30, 39, 49, 96, 106
Open seclusion 5, 112
Organization 21, 78, 82–3, 92, 117,
   123, 138–9, 173
Out-patient 130
Overcrowding 22, 104

Paternalism 129, 149, 153–6
Patient's Charter 30, 79–80
Personhood 151–2
Philosophy 2, 37 83, 93, 98–9,
   143–5, 146–60
Physical abuse 127–45
Pindown 6, 137
Pinel 18, 24, 27
Pink, Graham 119